# Contributions to Nephrology

**Vol. 187**

Series Editor

Claudio Ronco  Vicenza

**Acute Kidney Injury – From Diagnosis to Care**

# Acute Kidney Injury – From Diagnosis to Care

Volume Editors

**Xiaoqiang Ding** Shanghai
**Claudio Ronco** Vicenza

16 figures, 20 tables, 2016

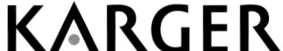

Basel · Freiburg · Paris · London · New York · Chennai · New Delhi ·
Bangkok · Beijing · Shanghai · Tokyo · Kuala Lumpur · Singapore · Sydney

**Contributions to Nephrology**

(Founded 1975 by Geoffrey M. Berlyne)

**Xiaoqiang Ding**
Division of Nephrology
Zhongshan Hospital
Shanghai Medical College
Fudan University
No. 180 Fenglin Road
CN–200032 Shanghai (China)

**Claudio Ronco**
Department of Nephrology
Dialysis and Transplantation
International Renal Research Institute
(IRRIV)
San Bortolo Hospital
Viale Rodolfi, 37
IT–36100 Vicenza (Italy)

Library of Congress Cataloging-in-Publication Data

Names: Ding, Xiaoqiang (Of Fu dan da xue (Shanghai, China)), editor. | Ronco,
  C. (Claudio), 1951- , editor.
Title: Acute kidney injury : from diagnosis to care / volume editors, Xiaoqiang Ding, Claudio Ronco.
Other titles: Acute kidney injury : from diagnosis to care (Ding) | Contributions to nephrology ; v.
  187. 0302-5144
Description: Basel ; New York : Karger, 2016. | Series: Contributions to
  nephrology, ISSN 0302-5144 ; vol. 187 | Includes bibliographical
  references and indexes.
Identifiers: LCCN 2015050912| ISBN 9783318058253 (hard cover : alk. paper) |
  ISBN 9783318058260 (e-ISBN)
Subjects: | MESH: Acute Kidney Injury | Kidney--injuries | Renal Replacement
  Therapy
Classification: LCC RC918.R4 | NLM WJ 342 | DDC 617.4/61044--dc23 LC record available at
  http://lccn.loc.gov/2015050912

Bibliographic Indices. This publication is listed in bibliographic services, including Current Contents® and Index Medicus.

Disclaimer. The statements, opinions and data contained in this publication are solely those of the individual authors and contributors and not of the publisher and the editor(s). The appearance of advertisements in the book is not a warranty, endorsement, or approval of the products or services advertised or of their effectiveness, quality or safety. The publisher and the editor(s) disclaim responsibility for any injury to persons or property resulting from any ideas, methods, instructions or products referred to in the content or advertisements.

Drug Dosage. The authors and the publisher have exerted every effort to ensure that drug selection and dosage set forth in this text are in accord with current recommendations and practice at the time of publication. However, in view of ongoing research, changes in government regulations, and the constant flow of information relating to drug therapy and drug reactions, the reader is urged to check the package insert for each drug for any change in indications and dosage and for added warnings and precautions. This is particularly important when the recommended agent is a new and/or infrequently employed drug.

All rights reserved. No part of this publication may be translated into other languages, reproduced or utilized in any form or by any means electronic or mechanical, including photocopying, recording, microcopying, or by any information storage and retrieval system, without permission in writing from the publisher.

© Copyright 2016 by S. Karger AG, P.O. Box, CH–4009 Basel (Switzerland)
www.karger.com
Printed in Germany on acid-free and non-aging paper (ISO 9706) by Kraft Druck, Ettlingen
ISSN 0302–5144
e-ISSN 1662–2782
ISBN 978–3–318–05825–3
e-ISBN 978–3–318–05826–0

# Contents

**VII Preface**
Ding, X. (Shanghai); Ronco, C. (Vicenza)

## AKI Characteristics and Epidemiology

**1 Acute Kidney Injury Epidemiology: From Recognition to Intervention**
Wang, Y.; Fang, Y.; Teng, J.; Ding, X. (Shanghai)

**9 Acute Kidney Injury Prevention**
Chopra, T.A.; Brooks, C.H.; Okusa, M.D. (Charlottesville, Va.)

**24 Renal Recovery after Acute Kidney Injury**
Macedo, E. (Sao Paulo); Mehta, R.L. (San Diego, Calif.)

## AKI Pathophysiology and Diagnosis

**36 Pathophysiology of Septic Acute Kidney Injury**
Mårtensson, J. (Melbourne, Vic./Stockholm); Bellomo, R. (Melbourne, Vic.)

**47 Biomarkers for Diagnosis, Prognosis and Intervention in Acute Kidney Injury**
Fuhrman, D.Y.; Kellum, J.A. (Pittsburgh, Pa.)

**55 The Acute Kidney Injury to Chronic Kidney Disease Transition: A Potential Opportunity to Improve Care in Acute Kidney Injury**
Palant, C.E.; Amdur, R.L.; Chawla, L.S. (Washington, D.C.)

**73 Electronic Data Systems and Acute Kidney Injury**
Cheungpasitporn, W.; Kashani, K. (Rochester, Minn.)

## AKI Management

**84 Fluid Management in Acute Kidney Injury**
Chuang, C.-L. (Taipei)

**94 Multidimensional Approach to Adequacy of Renal Replacement Therapy in Acute Kidney Injury**
Villa, G. (Florence); Ricci, Z. (Rome); Romagnoli, S. (Florence/Rome); Ronco, C. (Vicenza)

**106 Timing of Renal Replacement Therapy in Acute Kidney Injury**
Ostermann, M. (London); Wald, R. (Toronto, Ont.); Bagshaw, S.M. (Edmonton, Alta.)

**121 Pediatric Continuous Renal Replacement Therapy**
Ricci, Z. (Rome); Goldstein, S.L. (Cincinnati, Ohio)

**131 Management of Cardiac Surgery-Associated Acute Kidney Injury**
Xu, J.; Jiang, W.; Fang, Y.; Teng, J.; Ding, X. (Shanghai)

**143 Author Index**
**144 Subject Index**

# Preface

Once more, the book series Contributions to Nephrology is presenting a timely volume on one of the most intriguing and debated topics in the area of nephrology: acute kidney injury (AKI). The book is a compendium of contributions from the most renowned authors and AKI experts on all continents around the world.

The content is a synthetic yet complete review on the most controversial aspects of AKI, ranging from epidemiology and basic science to pathophysiology and clinical issues.

The book is intended to represent a good reference for physicians and nurses who deal with AKI in clinical nephrology and intensive care wards every day. The final result of this editorial effort is an updated compendium of state-of-the-art papers usable as a reference and a consultation tool for everyday clinical practice. The reader will benefit from the different contributions, treasuring the clear understanding and knowledge of the experts and applying these contributions to day-to-day practice.

The book should hopefully fill a gap in education and awareness of the importance of AKI and related issues. It should teach how a vision of the future and daily hard work together with a clear focus are the essential chemistry for diagnostic and therapeutic success. Many practices in medicine do not or cannot await for clinical trials to be supported by enough evidence but nevertheless are increasingly applied, with common acceptance of a tangible patient benefit. Only years after this vision came the demonstration of a significant benefit in survival for patients treated with specific AKI therapies. Thus, this book represents an important contribution to the field of AKI, offering students, young investigators and physicians the possibility to interact with worldwide experts not only through the existing evidence in the current literature but also through the vision of opinion leaders, which will pave the way toward future discoveries and clinical improvements.

*Xiaoqiang Ding*, Shanghai
*Claudio Ronco*, Vicenza

# Acute Kidney Injury Epidemiology: From Recognition to Intervention

Yimei Wang[a–d] · Yi Fang[a–d] · Jie Teng[a–d] · Xiaoqiang Ding[a–d]

[a]Division of Nephrology, Zhongshan Hospital, Shanghai Medical College, Fudan University, [b]Shanghai Institute for Kidney and Dialysis, [c]Key Laboratory of Kidney and Blood Purification of Shanghai, [d]Quality Control Center of Dialysis, Shanghai, China

## Abstract

Acute kidney injury (AKI) is very common among hospitalized patients, and the incidence of AKI has increased over the past few decades. This increase might be due to an aging population and increased comorbidities. Other factors that may explain this are the more sensitive diagnostic criteria and better recognition. AKI is associated with increased mortality and increased risks of chronic kidney disease and end-stage renal disease. The best ways to lower the chances of having kidney damage are to prevent, recognize and treat AKI as early as possible. The incidence of AKI in China is significantly lower than in developed countries. Inadequate early diagnosis and management remain the major challenges for Chinese nephrologists.

© 2016 S. Karger AG, Basel

Acute kidney injury (AKI) is an abrupt loss of kidney function. AKI was described for the first time by Galen (119–200) almost 2,000 years ago [1], but it did not have a consensus definition until a decade ago. AKI is a common and serious problem worldwide. The incidence of AKI is 3–20% in hospitalized patients and 30–60% in the intensive care unit (ICU) [2]. Nowadays, the mortality of AKI patients remains high, although great progress has been achieved in elucidating the mechanism and in performing renal replacement therapy (RRT) for AKI. AKI may lead to chronic kidney disease (CKD), regardless of the cause of AKI. To date, there is no specific treatment that increases survival in patients with or at high risk of AKI. The right therapy also includes the right timeframe, as delayed treatment sometimes has no benefit, so early recognition of AKI is especially important.

**Table 1.** Consensus definitions of AKI

| Definition | GFR | Serum creatinine | Urine output |
|---|---|---|---|
| RIFLE [2004] | Decrease >25% | Increase ≥50% from baseline, to be determined over 7 days | <0.5 ml/kg/h for 6 h |
| AKIN [2007] | – | Increase ≥0.3 mg/dl (26.4 µmol/l) or ≥50% within 48 h | <0.5 ml/kg/h for more than 6 h |
| KDIGO [2012] | – | Increase ≥0.3 mg/dl (26.4 µmol/l) within 48 h or ≥50% above baseline or presumed to have occurred within the prior 7 days | <0.5 ml/kg/h for 6 h |

RIFLE = Risk, Injury, Failure, Loss, and End-stage renal disease; AKIN = Acute Kidney Injury Network.

## Definition of Acute Kidney Injury

Before 2004, acute renal failure (ARF) was diagnosed based on an abrupt and sustained decrease in the glomerular filtration rate (GFR), resulting in retention of waste products. The lack of a precise definition of ARF resulted in more than 30 definitions in the medical literature [3], which caused wide variation in the reported incidence and clinical significance of ARF.

*'Risk, Injury, Failure, Loss, and End-Stage Renal Disease' Classification*
In 2004, the birth of the 'Risk, Injury, Failure, Loss, and End-stage renal disease' classification opened a new era for the definition of AKI [4] (table 1). This was the first consensus definition based on serum creatinine (SCr), the estimated GFR and urine output, which provided a platform through which comparative epidemiology could be judged. This classification greatly improved the early detection of AKI.

*Acute Kidney Injury Network*
In 2007, the AKI Network published their AKI criteria for adults, serving an evolution of the criteria outlined above [5] (table 1). The Risk, Injury, and Failure stages became stages 1, 2, and 3. A rise of ≥0.3 mg/dl in creatinine within 48 h was included in stage 1, which made the definition more sensitive. The GFR criterion was removed as a marker of AKI.

*Kidney Disease: Improving Global Outcomes*
In 2012, the Kidney Disease: Improving Global Outcomes (KDIGO) guidelines revised the AKI definition again [6] (table 1). KDIGO made one additional change to the criteria for the sake of simplicity: patients can reach stage 3 due to SCr >4.0 mg/dl (353.6 µmol/l), rather than requiring an acute increase of ≥0.5 mg/dl (44.2 µmol/l).

Many studies that evaluated these classification schemes have shown clear associations between the severity of AKI and poor outcomes. However, the current definitions of AKI are still not perfect.

The diagnosis of AKI depends on the baseline SCr, which is often unknown. If we use back-calculated SCr by reversing the 'Modification of Diet in Renal Disease' equation, with a normal GFR of 75 ml/min per 1.73 m$^2$ [7], the baseline SCr will often be underestimated, and false-positive detection of AKI will increase. Use of the admission SCr, thus ignoring preadmission AKI, underestimates the incidence of AKI.

SCr can be affected by age, gender, ethnicity, dietary protein intake, and muscle mass. In addition, following a critical illness, the patient with a long ICU stay often has a low SCr concentration due to muscle wasting and fluid overload. Meanwhile, urine output can be affected by diuretic use and volume status. Therefore, definitions based on these factors are not reliable enough. In the near future, novel kidney damage biomarkers may be added to the definition for early AKI diagnosis and prognosis prediction [8].

## High Incidence

The incidence of AKI has increased over the years. A recent meta-analysis showed that the pooled incidence of AKI is high across a worldwide spectrum [9]. The study examined 312 studies, with 95% from hospital settings and most from critical care. The incidence rates of AKI were 21.6% in adults and 33.7% in children. In a US study (n = 3,787,410), the community-based incidences of non-RRT-requiring AKI and RRT-requiring AKI were estimated at 384.1 and 24.4 per 100,000 person-years, respectively [10]. For 1992–2001 (5% sample of US hospitalized Medicare beneficiaries, n = 5,403,015), the incidence rate of AKI increased from 1.43 to 3.59%, with rates increasing by approximately 11% per year. The overall in-hospital death rate was 4.6% in AKI patients [11].

The AKI incidence in the ICU is extremely high, or 27–67% [12, 13]. The multinational AKI-EPI study enrolled 1,032 ICU patients from 97 centers in 33 countries and found that 57.3% patients suffered from AKI and that the adjusted incidence and mortality of AKI were similar worldwide (but none of the centers was in a low-income country). RRT was used in 13.5% of ICU patients (23.5% of patients with AKI). Sepsis and hypovolemia were the most common etiologies for AKI [14].

The rate of RRT-requiring AKI increased simultaneously. From 2000 to 2009, the incidence of dialysis-requiring AKI in the US increased from 222 to 533 cases per million person-years, averaging a 10% increase per year [15]. In a retrospective study of coronary artery bypass grafting patients (n = 7,339,520),

**Table 2.** Risk factors for AKI

| Non-modifiable | Modifiable |
| --- | --- |
| Advanced age | Anemia |
| Male gender | Sepsis |
| Black race | Fluid overload |
| Chronic kidney disease | Volume depletion |
| Hypertension | Nephrotoxic medications |
| Diabetes | Radio-contrast agents |
| Chronic diseases (heart, lung, liver, etc.) | Surgery |
| Cancer | |
| Hyperuricemia | |

the incidence of RRT-requiring AKIT increased from 0.2 to 0.6% from 1988 to 2003, respectively [16].

The higher incidence of AKI can be attributed to the following factors: (1) population aging: elderly people have a higher risk of AKI because of a decreased GFR and a diminished kidney reserve; (2) consensus definition: this resulted in more effective and simple diagnosis of AKI; (3) severe comorbidities: CKD, diabetes, hypertension and cardiovascular disease, the predominant preexisting risk factors for AKI, are increasing year by year [17]; (4) expansion of modifiable risk factors (sepsis, contrast agents, nephrotoxic drugs and surgery); and (5) E-alerting: an automated, real-time electronic alert system can improve early detection by providing advice on appropriate early management and timely referral to the nephrologist [18]. Risk factors for AKI are listed in table 2.

Few data on AKI epidemiology are from developing countries. It seems that AKI affects mainly young and previously healthy people in developing countries. The causes of AKI in developing countries differ from those in developed countries. The leading causes of AKI are infectious diseases (malaria, leptospirosis, dengue and diarrhea), obstetric diseases and toxic mechanisms (snake, spider and insect bites) [19].

*Community-Acquired Acute Kidney Injury and Hospital-Acquired Acute Kidney Injury*

Hospital-acquired AKI (HA-AKI) is defined as the development of AKI after 48 h of hospitalization. The most common causes of HA-AKI are acute tubular necrosis, sepsis, nephrotoxic medications and contrast nephropathy. Few studies have focused on community-acquired AKI (CA-AKI). A retrospective cohort analysis of New York Veterans Affairs hospitals revealed that CA-AKI was 3.5 times as prevalent as HA-AKI and had similar 3-year outcomes [20]. Among 15,976 hospitalized patients in the UK, the incidence of CA-AKI and HA-AKI was 4.3 and 2.1%, respectively, with CA-AKI patients having better short- and long-term outcomes [21].

## Poor Outcomes

*High Mortality*
Previous studies have described the independent association of AKI with a higher risk of death [2, 9]. The estimated unadjusted mortality of AKI is 23.9% in adults and 13.8% in children around the world [9]. The mortality rates increase with AKI stage. A study of patients who had undergone cardiac surgery (n = 3,245) found that the AKI incidence was 39.9% and that the 2-year overall survival rates of patients with AKI stages 1, 2, and 3 were 89.9, 78.6, and 61.4%, respectively [22]. The risk factors for mortality associated with AKI include acute myocardial infarction, acute heart failure, major noncardiac and cardiac surgeries, and critical illness. AKI also leads to a longer stay in the hospital, rehospitalization, worse quality of life and a huge social burden [23]. AKI was one of the most expensive diseases in US hospitals in 2011, with an aggregated cost of nearly USD 4.7 billion for about 498,000 hospital stays [24]. AKI is estimated to cost the UK National Health Service up to GBP 620 million every year [25]. What delights us is that AKI-associated mortality is decreasing. This is probably due to earlier diagnosis, more nephrology consultations and effective treatment [23].

*Progression to Chronic Kidney Disease and End-Stage Renal Disease*
Even if patients survive an episode of AKI, few of them are able to achieve complete recovery of renal function. Many AKI patients, and particularly the elderly and those with preexisting CKD, will progress to CKD and end-stage renal disease (ESRD) gradually. A systematic review and meta-analysis indicated that the pooled incidences of CKD and ESRD were 25.8 and 8.6 per 100 person-years, respectively [26]. Among 556,090 US patients, the 8-year risk of progressive CKD in patients with RRT-requiring AKI was found 28-fold greater than in non-AKI groups [27].

Renal recovery in AKI is currently being investigated, but there is still a lack of a consensus definition. A wide range of renal recovery rates have been reported, from 30 to 76%. The common renal recovery criteria are (1) a lack of RRT; (2) a return to within 50% of the baseline SCr; (3) a return to within 10–20% of the baseline SCr; (4) a return to within 10–20% of the baseline SCr; and (5) an estimated GFR >60 ml/min/1.73 m$^2$. Moreover, the definition of renal recovery should have a time point: hospital discharge, 28 days, 90 days or long-term prognosis [28]. Consensus agreement on meaningful definitions of recovery is needed, just like for AKI 10 years ago.

**Acute Kidney Injury in China**

China is a developing country with the largest population in the world. The epidemiological data on AKI in China have attracted increasing attention worldwide in the last decade. In 2015, a nationwide cross-sectional study from 44 hospitals in 22 provinces revealed that the incidence of AKI was 0.99% among 2,223,230 hospitalized patients according the KDIGO classification. The RRT rate and the in-hospital mortality were 14.4 and 12.4%, respectively [29]. Recent single-center studies have shown that AKI is a complicating factor in 2.4–8.1% of all hospital adult admissions and in up to 30–50% of ICU patients, with an associated mortality rate of 18.6–28.5% in those affected [30, 31]. It is estimated that 1.4–2.9 million people with AKI are admitted to the hospital in China per year, consuming about USD 13 billion for their in-hospital cost [29].

In large cities and university hospitals in China, the AKI spectrum is similar to that in developed countries. There are no reliable statistics on AKI in low-income areas. Venomous snake bites, organophosphorus pesticide/paraquat poisoning, bee stings and mushrooms and fish gut consumption lead to AKI in some rural areas. Aristolochic acid-associated nephropathy can occur in people who have consumed certain amounts of traditional Chinese herbs containing aristolochic acid [31].

In China, AKI is poorly recognized and managed. Only 25.8% AKI patients are identified, and renal referral is done in 21.4% of AKI cases, falling behind the rate in developed countries [31]. Awareness of AKI is urgently needed among nephrologists, surgeons, intensivists and other physicians in China.

**Acute Kidney Injury Is Preventable and Treatable**

Recently, the International Society of Nephrology has launched the '0 by 25' initiative to eliminate preventable deaths from AKI worldwide by 2025 [32]. The key elements in any AKI prevention strategy for hospitalized patients are to identify the patients with a high risk of AKI and to avoid hypovolemia and nephrotoxins. Intravenous saline therapy with or without additional sodium bicarbonate supplementation is the only recommended prophylaxis against contrast-induced AKI [2]. Recent evidence suggests that remote ischemic preconditioning, a novel inexpensive and noninvasive treatment, may prevent AKI, especially among patients undergoing cardiac surgery and contrast administration [33]. Recent studies with early nephrology consultation have shown a decrease in the incidence and severity of AKI. Timely nephrology referral can lead to appropriate prevention and intervention. A real-time electronic alert can provide identification of AKI patients, prompting therapy and better outcomes [18].

## Conclusions

AKI is now considered to be a major public health problem affecting millions of people worldwide and leading to increased mortality, a longer length of hospital stay and higher risks of CKD and ESRD. AKI is from communities and hospitals, with 95% of studies focused on the renal division. It is necessary to raise awareness of AKI among the public, government officials, and all health care professionals. The incidence and mortality of AKI both remain high, so future research should focus on improvement of the definitions of AKI, renal recovery and on novel interventions to improve AKI outcomes.

## Acknowledgment

We thank the National Clinical Key Subject Construction Projects, the Shanghai Health System Promotion Projects of Appropriate Use of Advanced Technology (2013SY048), and the Project of Technology Committee in Shanghai (12DJ1400200) for funding this work.

## References

1. Eknoyan G: The origins of nephrology – Galen, the founding father of experimental renal physiology. Am J Nephrol 1989;9:66–82.
2. Lameire NH, Bagga A, Cruz D, et al: Acute kidney injury: an increasing global concern. Lancet 2013;382:170–179.
3. Lameire N, Van Biesen W, Vanholder R: Acute renal failure. Lancet 2005;365:417–430.
4. Bellomo R, Ronco C, Kellum JA, et al: Acute renal failure definition, outcome measures, animal models, fluid therapy and information technology needs: the Second International Consensus Conference of the Acute Dialysis Quality Initiative (ADQI) Group. Crit Care 2004;8:R204–R212.
5. Mehta RL, Kellum JA, Shah SV, et al: Acute Kidney Injury Network: report of an initiative to improve outcomes in acute kidney injury. Crit Care 2007;11:R31.
6. Kidney Disease Improving Global Outcomes: KDIGO Clinical Practice Guideline for Acute Kidney Injury. Kidney Int 2012;2(suppl):8–12.
7. Bagshaw SM, Uchino S, Cruz D, et al: A comparison of observed versus estimated baseline creatinine for determination of RIFLE class in patients with acute kidney injury. Nephrol Dial Transplant 2009;24:2739–2744.
8. Legrand M, Darmon M: Biomarkers for AKI improve clinical practice: yes. Intensive Care Med 2015;41:615–617.
9. Susantitaphong P, Cruz DN, Cerda J, et al: World incidence of AKI: a meta-analysis. Clin J Am Soc Nephrol 2013;8:1482–1493.
10. Hsu CY, McCulloch CE, Fan D, et al: Community-based incidence of acute renal failure. Kidney Int 2007;72:208–212.

11 Xue JL, Daniels F, Star RA, et al: Incidence and mortality of acute renal failure in Medicare beneficiaries, 1992 to 2001. J Am Soc Nephrol 2006;17:1135–1142.
12 Bagshaw SM, George C, Bellomo R, et al: A comparison of the RIFLE and AKIN criteria for acute kidney injury in critically ill patients. Nephrol Dial Transplant 2008;23: 1569–1574.
13 Hoste EA, Clermont G, Kersten A, et al: RIFLE criteria for acute kidney injury are associated with hospital mortality in critically ill patients: a cohort analysis. Crit Care 2006; 10:R73.
14 Hoste EA, Bagshaw SM, Bellomo R, et al: Epidemiology of acute kidney injury in critically ill patients: the multinational AKI-EPI study. Intensive Care Med 2015;41:1411–1423.
15 Hsu RK, McCulloch CE, Dudley RA, et al: Temporal changes in incidence of dialysis-requiring AKI. J Am Soc Nephrol 2013;24: 37–42.
16 Nicoara A, Patel UD, Phillips-Bute BG, et al: Mortality trends associated with acute renal failure requiring dialysis after CABG surgery in the United States. Blood Purif 2009;28: 359–363.
17 Siew ED, Davenport A: The growth of acute kidney injury: a rising tide or just closer attention to detail? Kidney Int 2015;87:46–61.
18 Porter CJ, Juurlink I, Bisset LH, et al: A real-time electronic alert to improve detection of acute kidney injury in a large teaching hospital. Nephrol Dial Transplant 2014;29:1888–1893.
19 Cerdá J, Bagga A, Kher V, et al: The contrasting characteristics of acute kidney injury in developed and developing countries. Nat Clin Pract Nephrol 2008;4:138–153.
20 Der Mesropian PJ, Kalamaras JS, Eisele G, et al: Long-term outcomes of community-acquired versus hospital-acquired acute kidney injury: a retrospective analysis. Clin Nephrol 2014;81:174–184.
21 Wonnacott A, Meran S, Amphlett B, et al: Epidemiology and outcomes in community-acquired versus hospital-acquired AKI. Clin J Am Soc Nephrol 2014;9:1007–1014.
22 Xu JR, Zhu JM, Jiang J, et al: Risk factors for long-term mortality and progressive chronic kidney disease associated with acute kidney injury after cardiac surgery. Medicine (Baltimore) 2015;94:e2025.
23 Rewa O, Bagshaw SM: Acute kidney injury-epidemiology, outcomes and economics. Nat Rev Nephrol 2014;10:193–207.
24 Torio CM, Andrews RM: National Inpatient Hospital Costs: The Most Expensive Conditions by Payer, 2011: Statistical Brief #160 – Healthcare Cost and Utilization Project (HCUP) Statistical Briefs.
25 National Confidential Enquiry into Patient Outcome and Death: Adding Insult to Injury: A Review of the Care of Patients Who Died in Hospital with a Primary Diagnosis of Acute Kidney Injury (Acute Renal Failure). London, UK, NCEPOD, 2009.
26 Coca SG, Singanamala S, Parikh CR: Chronic kidney disease after acute kidney injury: a systematic review and meta-analysis. Kidney Int 2012;81:442–448.
27 Lo LJ, Go AS, Chertow GM, et al: Dialysis-requiring acute renal failure increases the risk of progressive chronic kidney disease. Kidney Int 2009;76:893–899.
28 Schortgen F: Defining renal recovery: pitfalls to be avoided. Intensive Care Med 2015;41: 1993–1995.
29 Yang L, Xing G, Wang L, et al: Acute kidney injury in China: a cross-sectional survey. Lancet 2015;386:1465–1471.
30 Fang Y, Ding X, Zhong Y, et al: Acute kidney injury in a Chinese hospitalized population. Blood Purif 2010;30:120–126.
31 Fang Y, Teng J, Ding X: Acute kidney injury in China. Hemodial Int 2015;19:2–10.
32 Mehta RL, Cerdá J, Burdmann EA, et al: International Society of Nephrology's 0by25 initiative for acute kidney injury (zero preventable deaths by 2025): a human rights case for nephrology. Lancet 2015;385:2543–2616.
33 Zarbock A, Milles K: Novel therapy for renal protection. Curr Opin Anaesthesiol 2015;28: 431–438.

Xiaoqiang Ding, MD, PhD
Division of Nephrology, Zhongshan Hospital
Shanghai Medical College, Fudan University
No.180 Fenglin Road, Shanghai 200032 (China)
E-Mail dingxiaoqiang2015@hotmail.com

# Acute Kidney Injury Prevention

Tushar A. Chopra · Charles H. Brooks · Mark D. Okusa

Division of Nephrology, Center for Immunity, Inflammation and Regenerative Medicine, University of Virginia, Charlottesville, Va., USA

## Abstract

Acute kidney injury (AKI) is a condition associated with significant morbidity and mortality. The incidence of AKI is increasing due to predisposing factors (sepsis, nephrotoxins, and hypotension). This review will focus on the risk stratification of patients vulnerable to developing AKI in whom the timing of the insult is known (e.g., cardiac surgery, contrast exposure) as well as the clinical context in which the risk intensifies. The review will also focus on preventive measures and different pharmacological agents for preventing AKI. Clinical trials of pharmacological agents for the prevention of AKI are challenging. While many compounds are promising in preclinical testing, only a few compounds have been tested, and none has shown consistent results in clinical trials. This is in part due to the lack of large and well-designed trials. With well-designed clinical trials, the use of novel biomarkers and innovative therapeutic strategies, we are on the verge of improving outcomes in the prevention of AKI.

© 2016 S. Karger AG, Basel

Acute kidney injury (AKI) is a serious medical condition that is defined by an abrupt decline in the glomerular filtration rate (GFR) over the course of hours to days and that is associated with abnormalities in fluid, electrolyte, acid-base and metabolic homeostasis. AKI was once considered a bystander that reflected other comorbidities, but it is now considered an independent risk factor for mortality [1]. The incidence of dialysis-requiring AKI is increasing, especially in the elderly [2]. The mortality rate continues to remain high, especially in the intensive care unit, but appears to be declining [3]. Consequently, in those patients who survive AKI and are discharged from the hospital, there is evidence that there is a marked increase in the risk of end-stage renal disease in severe dialysis-requiring AKI [4].

There are multiple causes of AKI and predisposing factors that likely contribute to the increased incidence of AKI. Despite preclinical studies demonstrating the efficacy of several promising interventions for the prevention of AKI, translation of these positive findings in preclinical studies to success in human AKI has been disappointing. To better understand failures in clinical trials, much attention has been focused on past clinical trial design [5]. In addition, recent attention has focused on preclinical animal studies, which often lack statistical rigor, randomization, sex heterogeneity, pharmacokinetic and pharmacodynamic studies and reporting of negative data, leading to publication bias [6]. Investigators, journals and the National Institutes of Health have raised these concerns to improve reproducibility and transparency in experimental studies.

This review will focus on (1) risk assessment to identify patients at high risk for AKI as prevention of AKI can best be achieved by minimizing exposure to high-risk subjects; (2) nonpharmacological interventions; and (3) past and novel pharmacological interventions. Thus, to prevent AKI, we need to identify patients at high risk for AKI, to prevent potential insults or to maximize protective strategies.

**Risk Assessment**

Assessing the risk of AKI in surgical procedures has been difficult due to changes in the definition of AKI and changes in outcomes-based reporting preferences, favoring information on the most severe forms of AKI or on those requiring dialysis. These observations were quantified in a study of 27,841 adult patients with no history of chronic kidney disease (CKD) who were undergoing major surgery [7]. Using the Kidney Disease: Improving Global Outcomes (KDIGO) criteria, there was a 37% incidence of AKI in this population, versus a 7% incidence using the National Surgical Quality Improvement Program criteria.

Risk assessment in high-risk cardiac surgery patients should focus not only on the factors significantly associated with AKI in major surgery but also on the clinical context. Thus, the following sections will address the risk of AKI in 3 areas of cardiovascular interventions: (1) conventional open procedures typically requiring cardio-pulmonary pump support, (2) transcatheter aortic valve replacement (TAVR), and (3) ventricular assist devices (VADs).

*Conventional Open Cardiac Surgery*
Demirjian conducted a prospective observational study examining presurgical and a combination of presurgical and intrasurgical variables in 25,898 patients undergoing cardiac surgery over an 8-year period to develop models predictive

**Table 1.** Factors for predicting AKI based on pre- and intrasurgical variables (p < 0.001)

| Doubling of serum creatinine or dialysis | Dialysis |
| --- | --- |
|  | Race |
| Body mass index |  |
|  | Pulmonary disease |
| Congestive heart failure |  |
| Diabetes mellitus |  |
| Emergent surgery | Emergent surgery |
| Estimated GFR | Estimated GFR |
| Albumin |  |
| Serum urea nitrogen | Serum urea nitrogen |
|  | Bilirubin |
| Cardio-pulmonary bypass time | Cardio-pulmonary bypass time |
| Intrasurgical packed RBC transfusions | Intrasurgical packed RBC transfusions |
| Intrasurgical vasopressor use | Intrasurgical vasopressor use |
| Intrasurgical urine output | Intrasurgical urine output |

RBC = Red blood cell.

of AKI. The incidence of AKI requiring dialysis was 1.7%, while the incidence of AKI represented by either dialysis or a doubling of the serum creatinine was 4.3%. Notably, the mortality rate for those requiring dialysis in this study was 48%, while in those with only a doubling of the serum creatinine, the mortality rate was 10% [8] (table 1). The authors compared the Cleveland Clinic risk score previously published by Thakar [9] to assess this cohort and found that it demonstrated excellent discrimination, with a C statistic of 0.843, but inadequate calibration.

*Transcatheter Aortic Valve Replacement*
TAVR is a therapeutic option for those severe aortic stenosis patients with unacceptable risks who are deemed ineligible for conventional open surgical aortic valve replacement (SAVR). Many studies have compared the outcomes of TAVR versus SAVR patients. In a 12-year single-center study of 2,169 patients undergoing SAVR, the incidence of AKI was 8.5% using the Acute Kidney Injury Network criteria and 3.9% using dialysis as the criterion [10]. By comparison, in a study of 102 TAVR patients [11], the incidence of AKI was 41.7% (Stage 1, 32.4%; Stage 2, 4.9%; and Stage 3, 3.9%). There was also access site variability in the incidence of AKI: among those with AKI, the incidence of AKI was 66.7% for trans-apical access, 30.3% for trans-femoral access, and 50% for trans-subclavian access. Trans-apical access was an independent predictor of AKI. A baseline GFR <30 ml/min and postprocedure Stage 3 AKI were independent predictors of 1-year mortality.

*Ventricular Assist Devices*
In a study of 53 patients with similar baseline characteristics who underwent VAD placement, 24 of the 53 patients developed AKI, versus 29 who did not. The patients who developed post-VAD AKI had a longer cardio-pulmonary bypass time; a greater need for re-operation; a higher risk of bleeding intraoperatively; and a higher incidence of infections, ventricular arrhythmias and right ventricular failure. Higher pre-VAD serum creatinine was associated with an increased risk of requiring dialysis. Lower survival rates were observed in the AKI group (hazard ratio 8.5) [12]. Further study of the incidence of AKI risk by stage relative to pre-left-VAD renal function would benefit the patient selection process.

Utilizing evidence to predict the risk of AKI in clinical practice informs clinical decision-making for patient selection, provides the basis for developing a multi-disciplinary risk reduction strategy, and lends credence to informed consent discussions with patients. Models of risk prediction are by definition formulaic, but AKI risk reduction is the product of careful nephrological assessment of all modifiable risks and treatment of the metabolic consequences of AKI.

*Contrast-Induced Acute Kidney Injury*
Table 2 presents the established risk factors for contrast-induced AKI (CI-AKI). Validated risk prediction models using patient and procedural risk factors to assess CI-AKI exists for patients undergoing percutaneous coronary intervention. In the Mehran risk model, the overall occurrence of CI-AKI in the development set of the score was 13.1% (range 7.5–57.3%, corresponding to low (<5) and high (>16) risk scores, respectively), and the rate of CI-AKI increased exponentially with an increasing risk score. In the validation data set, a high-risk score was strongly associated with CI-AKI (range 8.4–55.9%, corresponding to low and high risk scores, respectively) [13]. These models help in counseling patients about the risk of the procedure, selecting prophylactic interventions and characterizing patients in studies of CI-AKI.

## Nonpharmacological Means of Prevention of Acute Kidney Injury

*Prevention of Contrast-Induced Acute Kidney Injury*
The mechanisms of CI-AKI have been postulated to be medullary hypoxia, direct cytotoxicity to the tubules, and generation of reactive oxygen species. CI-AKI has been associated with increased mortality [14] and CKD [15]. Strategies to prevent CI-AKI include selection of low-risk contrast agents, volume expansion, and pharmacological therapy.

**Table 2.** Risk factors for CI-AKI

| Patient-related | Undetermined association |
|---|---|
| – Baseline kidney function or chronic kidney disease | – Intraarterial contrast administration |
| – Diabetes mellitus | – Anemia |
| – Heart failure | – Proteinuria |
| – Advanced age | – Liver disease |
| – Intravascular volume depletion | |
| – Concurrent nephrotoxins | |
| – Hemodynamic instability | |
| – Metabolic syndrome* | |
| – Prediabetes* | |
| – Hyperuricemia* | |
| **Procedure-related** | **Conflicting risk factors*** |
| – High-osmolar contrast medium | – ACEI |
| – Increased volume of contrast | – ARB |
| – Increased dose of iodine | – Renal transplantation |
| – Repeated sequential procedures | – Diabetes with normal renal function |

* Conflicting and newer risk factors [48–50]. ACEI = Angiotensin-converting enzyme inhibitor; ARB = angiotensin receptor blocker.

*Selection of Low-Risk Contrast Agents*

The first-generation compounds were hypertonic compared to plasma (osmolality of 1,500–1,800 mOsm/kg). The second-generation agents are ionic dimers or nonionic monomers of iodinated benzene rings. They are less hypertonic than the high-osmolar contrast media (HOCM; 600–850 mOsm/kg). The newer-generation contrast agent iodixanol is a nonionic dimer that is iso-osmolar to human serum but more viscous than previous agents. There are some concerns that viscosity may be an independent risk factor for CI-AKI.

A meta-analysis of 24 randomized studies suggests that in contrast to HOCM, low-osmolar contrast media (LOCM) are less nephrotoxic in the presence of preexisting kidney disease. There is continued debate about the superiority of LOCM versus iso-osmolar contrast media. Aspelin et al. [16] randomized 129 patients with CKD who underwent angiography and found that there was a lower incidence of CI-AKI with iso-osmolar contrast media compared to LOCM. A meta-analysis of 25 randomized controlled trials concluded that iodixanol did not significantly reduce the risk of CI-AKI compared to LOCM (relative risk (RR) 0.81, 95% CI 0.61–1.04). However, in a subgroup analysis, iodixanol reduced risk significantly when compared to iohexol (RR 0.45, 95% CI 0.26–0.76; $p < 0.01$). When iodixanol was compared to other nonionic LOCM, the reduc-

**Table 3.** Summary of fluids in CI-AKI

| Avoid | Allow |
|---|---|
| – Hypotonic fluids (half normal saline) | – LVEDP-guided fluid administration |
| – Oral hydration | – Volume expansion with normal saline or isotonic sodium bicarbonate |
| – Forced euvolemic diuresis [51] | |
| – Unclear benefit for RenalGuard system | |

LVEDP = Left ventricular end-diastolic pressure.

tion in CI-AKI risk was not statistically significant (RR 0.97, 95% CI 0.72–1.32; p = 0.86) [17]. These findings suggest that iohexol may be a higher-risk agent for CI-AKI compared to other nonionic LOCM.

In summary, the KDIGO guidelines of 2012 recommend using 'either iso-osmolar or low-osmolar contrast media, rather than high-osmolar iodinated contrast media in patients at increased risk of CI-AKI'.

*Isotonic Saline versus Bicarbonate-Based Solutions*
Volume expansion offers renal protection against CI-AKI. Volume expansion with either normal saline (NS) or isotonic sodium bicarbonate at an infusion rate of 1–1.5 ml/kg/h for at least 6 h peri-procedural administration of contrast is recommended [18]. Oral hydration and use of half NS are not effective [19]. There remains clinical equipoise on the effectiveness of NS versus sodium bicarbonate as the fluid of choice. Table 3 summarizes different fluid administration strategies to prevent CI-AKI.

Merten et al. demonstrated the benefit of sodium bicarbonate in a single-center randomized controlled trial [20]. In total, 119 cardiac patients with a serum creatinine of 1.1 mg/dl were randomized to receive isotonic NS or sodium bicarbonate solution. The primary endpoint was defined as an increase in serum creatinine >25% within 48 h. The study was terminated early, as the incidence of CI-AKI was significantly lower in the bicarbonate group compared to the isotonic saline group (1.7 vs. 13.6%, p = 0.016). However, this study may have been flawed due to a type 1 error. If one additional patient from the bicarbonate group had developed CI-AKI, the results would not have been statistically significant.

A number of systematic reviews and meta-analyses comparing intravenous bicarbonate and intravenous saline and demonstrating inconsistent results have been published [21].

The Poseidon trial included 400 patients at high risk for CI-AKI undergoing coronary angiography [22]. The patients were randomized to either the control arm (0.9% NS 1 h before and 4 h after cardiac catheterization) or the intervention arm (the same 1 h pre-NS dose, but NS given postcatheterization based on left ventricular end-diastolic pressure). The strategy was to maximize fluid administration while minimizing volume overload to prevent CI-AKI. The patients in the intervention arm took up more fluid and had a reduction in CI-AKI from 16 to 7% compared to the control group but also received more fluid. The conclusion was that patients who are at high risk for CI-AKI need significant volume expansion to prevent CI-AKI.

*N-Acetyl Cysteine in Contrast-Induced Acute Kidney Injury*
N-Acetyl cysteine (NAC) is a thiol-containing antioxidant that has been used to reduce AKI in patients with acetaminophen-induced liver injury [23] as well as to ameliorate ischemic AKI in animal models [24]. The potential free-radical-scavenging function of NAC has led to several prevention trials for AKI.

Tepel conducted the first randomized trial with 83 patients undergoing computed tomography, who were administered 600 mg NAC or placebo for 2 days. The incidence of CI-AKI was significantly lower in the NAC group compared to the placebo group (2 vs. 21%, p = 0.01) [25]. Subsequently, many underpowered clinical trials and meta-analyses studied the efficacy of NAC, with mixed results [26].

The largest randomized, double-blinded, placebo-controlled trial was conducted by Berwanger et al. [27]. The Acetylcysteine for Contrast-induced nephropathy Trial (ACT) randomized 2,308 patients to receive 1,200 mg NAC or placebo orally twice daily for 2 days. The primary study endpoint was defined as an increase in serum creatinine by 25% at 48–96 h after angiography. There was no difference in the incidence of CI-AKI in the NAC versus the placebo arms (12.7 vs. 12.7%, p = 0.97). Additionally, a subgroup analysis of 367 patients with baseline serum creatinine of >1.5 mg/dl demonstrated no benefit of NAC in reducing 30-day mortality or the need for dialysis. Although a large sample size was studied and serious 30-day outcomes were evaluated, the trial had some deficiencies: 1) the baseline mean estimated GFR was only 70 ml/min/1.73 m$^2$, and only 15.7% patients had a serum creatinine of >1.5 mg/dl; 2) more than 20% of the procedures utilized HOCM; 3) the baseline serum creatinine was obtained up to 90 days preprocedure; and 4) no standardization of peri-procedural fluid management was performed.

Although the ACT trial suggests that NAC does not prevent small increases in serum creatinine or in serious 30-day outcomes in low-risk patients, there remains clinical equipoise on the use of NAC for the prevention of CI-AKI.

There are several limitations in NAC studies, such as variable definitions of CI-AKI, marked heterogeneity and small sample sizes. The impact of NAC on 'hard' patient outcomes, such as the need for renal replacement therapy, all-cause mortality, or doubling of serum creatinine, is rarely studied.

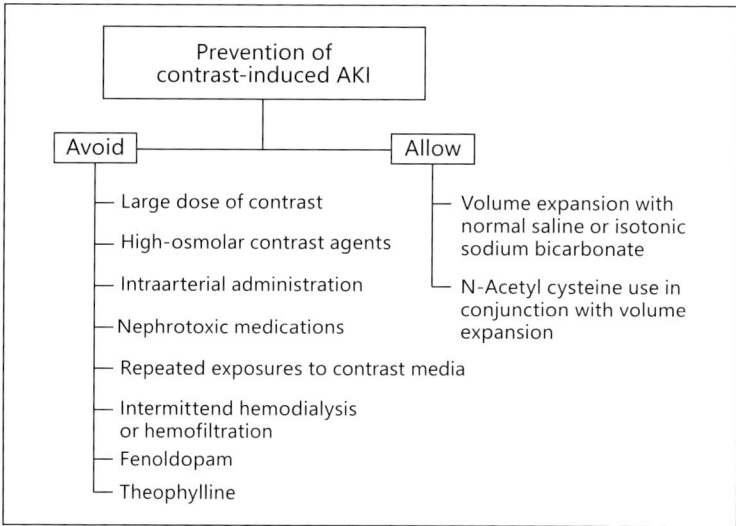

**Fig. 1.** Summary of prevention strategies for contrast-induced acute kidney injury [1].

As a result, the 2012 KDIGO guidelines suggest that oral NAC can be used along with isotonic crystalloids in patients with an increased risk of CI-AKI. However, the 2011 American College of Cardiology/American Heart Association guidelines suggest that NAC is not useful for the prevention of CI-AKI.

CI-AKI summary (fig. 1):

a. Use the lowest dose of contrast media.

b. Use either LOCM or iso-osmolar contrast media in conjunction with intravenous fluids, but avoid HOCM.

c. The risk of CI-AKI is greater for the intraarterial route compared to the intravenous route.

d. Administration of contrast media should be delayed in patients with circulatory collapse or congestive heart failure until their hemodynamic status is corrected.

e. Repeated exposure should be delayed for 48 h in patients without risk factors or for 72 h in patients with risk factors for CI-AKI with diabetes mellitus or preexisting CKD.

f. Concurrent nephrotoxic medications should be stopped.

g. There exists clinical equipoise on the comparative effectiveness of NS and bicarbonate-based solutions for the prevention of CI-AKI.

h. Intravenous volume expansion with either isotonic sodium chloride or sodium bicarbonate is recommended in patients with an increased risk of CI-AKI.

i. Prophylactic intermittent hemodialysis and hemofiltration should not be used for contrast media removal in patients at increased risk for CI-AKI.

**Prevention of Nephrotoxin-Induced Acute Kidney Injury**

Despite a number of clinical trials using different pharmacological agents for the prevention or treatment of AKI, there are no Food and Drug Administration-approved drugs for this condition (table 4). For the reasons described above, concerning patients with significant comorbidities, the complexity of AKI, the systemic nature of AKI, clinical trial design, the reproducibility of preclinical studies and the use of creatinine as a biomarker of AKI, these studies yielded negative results.

A classic example that illustrates the problems associated with the translation of preclinical studies to successful treatment of human AKI is the use of recombinant human insulin-like growth factor-I (rhIGF-I) for the treatment of AKI. In preclinical studies, rhIGF-I reduced kidney injury when administered 30 min after reperfusion in experimental ischemia-reperfusion injury (IRI) [28]. However, rhIGF-I failed to attenuate AKI in a human trial [29]. Confounding variables that were associated with rhIGF-I treatment included hypotension associated with rhIGF-I (42 vs. 27%) and treatment delay by as much as 6 days after diagnosis [29]. The efficacy of rhIGF-I in the prevention or treatment of AKI will likely remain unknown, as additional trials are likely not forthcoming. A similar argument can be made for the drugs listed in table 4, which will not be discussed further. Rather, we will focus on potential new drugs/compounds that are topical and of potential interest.

**Novel Targets for the Prevention of Acute Kidney Injury**

*Mitochondria-Targeted Antioxidants*
The mitochondria-targeted antioxidant mitoquinone mesylate (MitoQ) selectively accumulates in the mitochondrial matrix due to this antioxidant's positive charge. In the mitochondrial matrix, MitoQ is reduced to the active antioxidant form ubiquinol by the respiratory chain, thus protecting the tissue from lipid peroxidation and oxidative damage [30]. Administering MitoQ to mice intravenously 15 min prior to ischemia protects the kidney from damage and dysfunction.

SS-31 is a member of the Szeto-Schiller peptides that binds selectively to cardiolipin. Cardiolipin is a phospholipid that is expressed in the inner mitochondrial membrane and has an important structural role in the organization of respiratory complexes, allowing for efficient oxidative phosphorylation. Normal physiological interaction between cardiolipin and cytochrome *c* determines the fate of cytochrome *c* as an electron carrier or peroxidase. During AKI, it is

**Table 4.** Pharmacological interventions for preventing AKI (none approved by Food and Drug Administration)

| Drug | Mechanism | Therapeutic role |
|---|---|---|
| Vasopressors Dopamine (DA) Fenoldopam | Low-dose DA causes renal vasodilation, natriuresis, and an increased GFR | Studies have shown that DA significantly increased vascular resistance in patients with AKI, without any benefit for the prevention of AKI |
| | Fenoldopam is a selective DA type 1 receptor agonist | Although small studies suggested that fenoldopam can prevent AKI after cardiac surgery, a larger randomized controlled trial proved that it is ineffective in preventing AKI after cardiac surgery |
| Loop diuretics | Reduce tubular oxygen demand | Prophylactic use is harmful in AKI after cardiac surgery, and diuretics in CI-AKI do not reduce the incidence or severity of AKI |
| | Medullary wash out | Additionally, no significant reduction of renal replacement therapy requirement or in-hospital mortality |
| Mannitol | Dilutes nephrotoxins and maintains urine output via osmotic diuresis | Detrimental effect in CI-AKI; preventive administration just before clamp release may help to reduce posttransplant AKI, but no difference in kidney function was found at 3 months; adequately powered randomized controlled trials are lacking |
| Natriuretic peptides | Systemic renal vasodilators Enhance salt and water excretion | Prophylactic atrial natriuretic peptide has failed to prevent AKI |
| Anti-tumor lysis syndrome (TLS) agents Rasburicase Allopurinol | Lowers uric acid levels | Rasburicase effectively lowers uric acid levels and is more effective than allopurinol in preventing laboratory TLS, but rasburicase has not been shown to be more effective than allopurinol in preventing clinical TLS |
| Endothelin antagonist | Renal vasodilator | Not recommended for prophylaxis |
| Adenosine antagonist | Ameliorate tubuloglomerular feedback-mediated renal vasoconstriction in early ischemic acute tubular necrosis | Only indicated as a single renoprotective dose to prevent AKI stemming from perinatal asphyxia in neonates, but not beneficial for preventing AKI in adults |
| Statins | Pleiotropic effect, offering renal protection | Several positive studies demonstrated a protective effect against CI-AKI (TRACK-D trial), but most studies were prone to the 'healthy user effect' |

TRACK-D = Rosuvastatin Prevent Contrast Induced Acute Kidney Injury in Patients with Diabetes.

thought that this interaction is disrupted and that cytochrome *c* functions as a peroxidase. The interaction between SS-31 and cardiolipin through favorable electrostatic charges stabilizes cytochrome *c* and restores electron transport [31].

*Hypoxia-Inducible Factor Pathway*
Hypoxia-inducible factor (HIF) is a basic helix-loop-helix transcription factor that consists of the oxygen-sensitive α subunit HIF-α and the constitutively expressed β subunit HIF-β. Under normoxic conditions, a specific prolyl-hydroxylase (PHD) leads to the degradation of the HIF-α subunit through its hydroxylation and rapid proteasomal degradation by the von Hippel-Lindau tumor suppressor. Under hypoxic conditions, HIF-α is not degraded and translocates to the nucleus. There, it dimerizes with HIF-β, yielding a transcriptionally active HIF that regulates biological processes important for adaptation to oxygen deprivation. HIF-regulated genes include (but are not limited to) genes that are involved in glucose uptake and energy metabolism, angiogenesis, erythropoiesis, cell proliferation and apoptosis, cell-cell and cell-matrix interactions, and barrier function. HIF-2α activation results in the release of erythropoietin, which, in addition to its known ability to induce erythropoiesis, is also a cytoprotective molecule. PHD1 inhibitors inhibit endothelial HIF-2, which appears to be important in protecting against AKI [32]. Ongoing clinical trials are focused on PHD1 inhibitors (ClinicalTrials.gov).

*Peroxisome Proliferator-Activated Receptor-α Agonists*
Peroxisome proliferator-activated receptor-α (PPARα) is a member of the nuclear receptor superfamily of ligand-dependent transcription factors related to retinoid, steroid, and thyroid hormone receptors [33]. Fibrates are ligands for PPARα receptors that have been shown to have antiinflammatory properties. They have known effects on classically activated macrophages, blocking activator protein-1 and nuclear factor-κB signaling and inhibiting proinflammatory molecules, including interferon-gamma and interleukin-17. In animal models of AKI, fibrates protect from cisplatin-induced AKI [34] by preventing proximal tubule cell death.

*Bone Morphogenic Protein-7*
Bone morphogenic proteins (BMPs) are a family of proteins that belong to the transforming growth factor-β superfamily, which regulates cell growth, differentiation, and apoptosis and tissue repair [35]. BMPs signal through the SMAD pathway. Upon phosphorylation, SMADs are rapidly translocated to the cell nucleus through their association with SMAD4 [36]. When recombinant osteo-

genic protein-1 (BMP-7) was administered 10 min before or 1 or 16 h after bilateral renal artery occlusion, this protein reduced infarction, cellular necrosis, inflammation apoptosis and improved renal function [36]. THR-184 (Thrasos Innovation, Inc.), an agonist of the BMP pathway, is being tested in a clinical trial (NCT01830920, clinicaltrials.gov).

*Hepcidin-Ferroportin*
Catalytic iron ($Fe^{2+}$) is capable of catalyzing the Fenton and Haber-Weiss reactions, characterized by the interaction of superoxide anion ($O_2^-$) and hydrogen peroxide ($H_2O_2$), leading to the generation of hydroxyl radicals ($OH^-$) that cause oxidant tissue injury [37]. Evidence that catalytic iron contributes to nephrotoxicity comes from studies in which iron chelation attenuated injury in various animal models of AKI [38]. Recent studies have led to clarification of the molecular basis of iron trafficking, providing an opportunity to develop more specific compounds that target this pathway. $Fe^{2+}$ is exported from cells by ferroportin, an iron export protein that is expressed on macrophages, hepatocytes, renal proximal and distal tubular cells and enterocytes [39]. The endogenous peptide hormone hepcidin is primarily produced by hepatocytes [39] and is thought to bind to ferroportin, leading to its internalization and lysosomal degradation and thereby preventing cellular iron egress [40] and tissue injury. When infused into mice prior to IRI, hepcidin reduced inflammation and renal IRI [41]. The mechanism of protection is likely sequestration of catalytic iron through hepcidin's effects on decreasing kidney ferroportin expression and iron efflux and increasing the expression of cytoprotective H-ferritin [42]. These results suggest that targeting the hepcidin-ferroportin pathway may be effective in the treatment of AKI.

*Cell-Based Therapies*
Cell-based therapies affect innate immunity by targeting multiple sites. Mesenchymal stem cells (MSCs) generated from bone marrow can differentiate into osteocytes, chondrocytes and adipocytes. In various models of AKI (cisplatin-, glycerol- and IRI-induced), infused MSCs have been shown to have protective effects and to enhance recovery [43].

The contribution of transdifferentiated MSCs is low, but the tissue-protective effects are thought to be due to the production of growth factors and cytokines that modulate mitogenesis, apoptosis, and inflammation as well as vasculogenesis and angiogenesis. Additionally, microvesicles derived from MSCs have been shown to shuttle mRNA to injured cells to enhance survival [44]. Other forms of cell-based therapies may be useful in AKI, including regulatory $CD4^+CD25^+$ T cells (regulatory T cells) [45] or dendritic cells (DCs) [46]. DCs were tolerized by adenosine 2a agonist treatment, which attenuated kidney IRI [46]. Tolerized DCs can be generated through treatment with growth factors and cytokines as well as by genetic engineering and pharmacological agents [17].

## Conclusion

Core strategies to prevent AKI include close surveillance of at-risk patients; avoidance of nephrotoxic agents; and aiming to maintain adequate volume expansion, mean arterial pressure, and cardiac output. Prophylactic intravenous fluid therapy is an effective step in decreasing the risk of AKI. The majority of the prevention trials for AKI were not adequately powered, resulting in varying recommendations. Many successful preclinical results for compounds have yet to be reproduced in larger clinical studies to evaluate the compounds' role in preventing AKI. Emphasis should be placed on well-powered studies analyzing clinically relevant endpoints, e.g., long-term survival, and easily reproducible and measurable biomarkers and eliminating as many confounding variables as possible to yield meaningful results. Many novel preclinical targets may yield new therapeutic strategies for the prevention of AKI.

### References

1 Levy EM, Viscoli CM, Horwitz RI: The effect of acute renal failure on mortality. A cohort analysis. JAMA 1996;275:1489–1494.
2 Hsu RK, McCulloch CE, Dudley RA, et al: Temporal changes in incidence of dialysis-requiring AKI. J Am Soc Nephrol 2013;24: 37–42.
3 Waikar SS, Curhan GC, Wald R, et al: Declining mortality in patients with acute renal failure, 1988 to 2002. J Am Soc Nephrol 2006; 17:1143–1150.
4 Coca SG, Singanamala S, Parikh CR: Chronic kidney disease after acute kidney injury: a systematic review and meta-analysis. Kidney Int 2012;81:442–448.
5 Molitoris BA, Okusa MD, Palevsky PM, et al: Design of Clinical Trials in AKI: A Report from an NIDDK Workshop. Trials of Patients with Sepsis and in Selected Hospital Settings. Clin J Am Soc Nephrol 2012;7:856–860.
6 de Caestecker M, Humphreys BD, Liu KD, et al: Bridging translation by improving preclinical study design in AKI. J Am Soc Nephrol 2015, in press.
7 Bihorac A, Brennan M, Ozrazgat-Baslanti T, et al: National surgical quality improvement program underestimates the risk associated with mild and moderate postoperative acute kidney injury. Crit Care Med 2013;41:2570–2583.
8 Demirjian S, Schold JD, Navia J, et al: Predictive models for acute kidney injury following cardiac surgery. Am J Kidney Dis 2012;59: 382–389.
9 Thakar CV, Arrigain S, Worley S, et al: A clinical score to predict acute renal failure after cardiac surgery. J Am Soc Nephrol 2005; 16:162–168.
10 Najjar M, Yerebakan H, Sorabella RA, et al: Acute kidney injury following surgical aortic valve replacement. J Card Surg 2015;30:631–639.

11 Saia F, Ciuca C, Taglieri N, et al: Acute kidney injury following transcatheter aortic valve implantation: incidence, predictors and clinical outcome. In J Cardiol 2013;168:1034–1040.
12 Alba AC, Rao V, Ivanov J, et al: Predictors of acute renal dysfunction after ventricular assist device placement. J Card Fail 2009;15:874–881.
13 Mehran R, Aymong ED, Nikolsky E, et al: A simple risk score for prediction of contrast-induced nephropathy after percutaneous coronary intervention: development and initial validation. J Am Coll Cardiol 2004;44:1393–1399.
14 Weisbord SD, Chen H, Stone RA, et al: Associations of increases in serum creatinine with mortality and length of hospital stay after coronary angiography. J Am Soc Nephrol 2006;17:2871–2877.
15 James MT, Hemmelgarn BR, Wiebe N, et al: Glomerular filtration rate, proteinuria, and the incidence and consequences of acute kidney injury: a cohort study. Lancet 2010;376:2096–2103.
16 Aspelin P, Aubry P, Fransson SG, et al: Nephrotoxic effects in high-risk patients undergoing angiography. N Engl J Med 2003;348:491–499.
17 Heinrich MC, Haberle L, Muller V, et al: Nephrotoxicity of iso-osmolar iodixanol compared with nonionic low-osmolar contrast media: meta-analysis of randomized controlled trials. Radiology 2009;250:68–86.
18 Lameire N, Kellum JA, Group KAGW: Contrast-induced acute kidney injury and renal support for acute kidney injury: a KDIGO summary (Part 2). Crit Care 2013;17:205.
19 Trivedi HS, Moore H, Nasr S, et al: A randomized prospective trial to assess the role of saline hydration on the development of contrast nephrotoxicity. Nephron Clin Pract 2003;93:C29–C34.
20 Merten GJ, Burgess WP, Gray LV, et al: Prevention of contrast-induced nephropathy with sodium bicarbonate: a randomized controlled trial. JAMA 2004;291:2328–2334.
21 Brar SS, Hiremath S, Dangas G, et al: Sodium bicarbonate for the prevention of contrast induced-acute kidney injury: a systematic review and meta-analysis. Clin J Am Soc Nephrol 2009;4:1584–1592.
22 Brar SS, Aharonian V, Mansukhani P, et al: Haemodynamic-guided fluid administration for the prevention of contrast-induced acute kidney injury: the POSEIDON randomised controlled trial. Lancet 2014;383:1814–1823.
23 Brady HR, Singer GG: Acute renal failure. Lancet 1995;346:1533–1540.
24 DiMari J, Megyesi J, Udvarhelyi N, et al: N-acetyl cysteine ameliorates ischemic renal failure. Am J Physiol 1997;272:F292–F298.
25 Tepel M, van der Giet M, Schwarzfeld C, et al: Prevention of radiographic-contrast-agent-induced reductions in renal function by acetylcysteine. N Engl J Med 2000 Jul 20;343:180–184.
26 Weisbord SD, Gallagher M, Kaufman J, et al: Prevention of Contrast-Induced AKI: a review of published trials and the design of the prevention of serious adverse events following angiography (PRESERVE) trial. Clin J Am Soc Nephrol 2013;8:1618–1631.
27 ACT Investigators: Acetylcysteine for prevention of renal outcomes in patients undergoing coronary and peripheral vascular angiography: main results from the randomized Acetylcysteine for Contrast-induced nephropathy Trial (ACT). Circulation 2011;124:1250–1259.
28 Miller SB, Martin DR, Kissane J, et al: Insulin-like growth factor I accelerates recovery from ischemic acute tubular necrosis in the rat. Proc Natl Acad Sci U S A 1992;89:11876–11880.
29 Hirschberg R, Kopple J, Lipsett P, et al: Multicenter clinical trial of recombinant human insulin-like growth factor I in patients with acute renal failure. Kidney Int 1999;55:2423–2432.
30 Dare AJ, Bolton EA, Pettigrew GJ, et al: Protection against renal ischemia-reperfusion injury in vivo by the mitochondria targeted antioxidant MitoQ. Redox Biol 2015;5:163–168.
31 Szeto HH: First-in-class cardiolipin-protective compound as a therapeutic agent to restore mitochondrial bioenergetics. B J Pharmacol 2014;171:2029–2050.
32 Kapitsinou PP, Sano H, Michael M, et al: Endothelial HIF-2 mediates protection and recovery from ischemic kidney injury. J Clin Invest 2014;124:2396–2409.
33 Wang K, Wan YJ: Nuclear receptors and inflammatory diseases. Exp Biol Med 2008;233:496–506.

34 Li S, Gokden N, Okusa MD, et al: Anti-inflammatory effect of fibrate protects from cisplatin-induced ARF. Am J Physiol Renal Physiol 2005;289:F469–F480.
35 Lee SY, Kim SI, Choi ME: Therapeutic targets for treating fibrotic kidney diseases. Transl Res 2015;165:512–530.
36 Vukicevic S, Basic V, Rogic D, et al: Osteogenic protein-1 (bone morphogenetic protein-7) reduces severity of injury after ischemic acute renal failure in rat. J Clin Invest 1998;102:202–214.
37 Jacob AK, Hotchkiss RS, DeMeester SL, et al: Endothelial cell apoptosis is accelerated by inorganic iron and heat via an oxygen radical dependent mechanism. Surgery 1997;122:243–253; discussion 254.
38 Baliga R, Ueda N, Walker PD, et al: Oxidant mechanisms in toxic acute renal failure. Drug Metab Rev 1999;31:971–997.
39 Moulouel B, Houamel D, Delaby C, et al: Hepcidin regulates intrarenal iron handling at the distal nephron. Kidney Int 2013;84:756–766.
40 Nemeth E: Targeting the hepcidin-ferroportin axis in the diagnosis and treatment of anemias. Adv Hematol 2010;2010:1–9.
41 Scindia Y, Dey P, Thirunagari A, et al: Hepcidin mitigates renal ischemia-reperfusion injury by modulating systemic iron homeostasis. J Am Soc Nephrol 2015;26:2800–2814.
42 Zarjou A, Bolisetty S, Joseph R, et al: Proximal tubule H-ferritin mediates iron trafficking in acute kidney injury. J Clin Invest 2013;123:4423–4434.
43 Togel FE, Westenfelder C: Mesenchymal stem cells: a new therapeutic tool for AKI. Nat Rev Nephrol 2010;6:179–183.
44 Bruno S, Grange C, Deregibus MC, et al: Mesenchymal stem cell-derived microvesicles protect against acute tubular injury. J Am Soc Nephrol 2009;20:1053–1067.
45 Kinsey GR, Sharma R, Huang L, et al: Regulatory T cells suppress innate immunity in kidney ischemia-reperfusion injury. J Am Soc Nephrol 2009;20:1744–1753.
46 Li L, Huang L, Ye H, et al: Dendritic cells tolerized with adenosine A(2)AR agonist attenuate acute kidney injury. J Clin Invest 2012;122:3931–3942.
47 Morelli AE, Thomson AW: Tolerogenic dendritic cells and the quest for transplant tolerance. Nat Rev Immunol 2007;7:610–621.
48 Toprak O: Conflicting and new risk factors for contrast induced nephropathy. J Urol 2007;178:2277–2283.
49 Mehran R, Nikolsky E: Contrast-induced nephropathy: definition, epidemiology, and patients at risk. Kidney Int Suppl 2006;100:S11–S15.
50 McCullough PA, Adam A, Becker CR, et al: Risk prediction of contrast-induced nephropathy. Am J Cardiol 2006;98:27K–36K.
51 Majumdar SR, Kjellstrand CM, Tymchak WJ, et al: Forced euvolemic diuresis with mannitol and furosemide for prevention of contrast-induced nephropathy in patients with CKD undergoing coronary angiography: a randomized controlled trial. Am J Kidney Dis 2009;54:602–609.

Tushar A. Chopra, MD
Box 133, Division of Nephrology
University of Virginia Health Sciences Center
Charlottesville, VA 22908 (USA)
E-Mail TAC5V@hscmail.mcc.virginia.edu

# Renal Recovery after Acute Kidney Injury

Etienne Macedo[a] · Ravindra L. Mehta[b]

[a]Division of Nephrology, University of Sao Paulo, Sao Paulo, Brazil; [b]Division of Nephrology and Hypertension, Department of Medicine, University of California San Diego, San Diego, Calif., USA

## Abstract

Until recently, patients surviving an episode of acute kidney injury (AKI) were assumed to have a good renal prognosis. This belief was predominantly based on studies that used heterogeneous AKI definitions and that considered renal recovery as dialysis independence at hospital discharge. Since standardized definitions of AKI have become available, several studies have established an association between AKI and adverse clinical outcomes. It is now well recognized that while the glomerular filtration rate generally improves after AKI, the renal recovery process is often incomplete and can result in a chronic decrease in kidney function. The loss of kidney function can vary from subclinical decreases in the glomerular filtration rate to end-stage renal disease. In this chapter, we review our current understanding of renal recovery following AKI and discuss the main studies that have established associations between AKI and the development of chronic kidney disease and end-stage renal disease [1].

© 2016 S. Karger AG, Basel

Remarkable improvements in acute kidney injury (AKI) epidemiology have been achieved during the last decade using the Risk, Injury, Failure, Loss of kidney function, and End-stage kidney disease (RIFLE)/Acute Kidney Injury Network guidelines and, more recently, the Kidney Disease: Improving Global Outcomes (KDIGO) classification system [2–4]. Although studies have confirmed that most survivors of an AKI episode will become independent of renal replacement therapy (RRT) within a year, it has also become clear that a significant number of AKI survivors will develop chronic kidney disease (CKD) and that some will progress to end-stage renal disease (ESRD) [1, 5–10]. However, a lack of a consistent definition for recovery is partially responsible for the wide variation in kidney recovery reported in the recent literature, ranging from less than 1% to greater than 40% [11–14]. As a result, several factors influencing short- and long-term kidney outcomes have not been thoroughly evaluated and are not currently understood. Patient demographic characteristics, the clinical course of AKI, and factors associated with the process of care for these patients may all influence patient and kidney outcomes [2, 15–17]. In this chapter, we review epidemiologic studies on renal recovery from AKI and the current knowledge of patient characteristics and process-of-care factors that may influence the renal prognosis after AKI.

**How to Assess Renal Recovery**

The use of a standardized AKI definition brought considerable advances in the knowledge of AKI epidemiology. The use of the RIFLE and Acute Kidney Injury Network guidelines and, more recently, the KDIGO classification system has helped to strengthen the concept that even mild alterations in renal function can be responsible for increased morbidity and mortality. The progression to CKD and ESRD after an episode of AKI has become an important short- and long-term outcome, and more attention has been focused on the lack of complete renal recovery after an episode of AKI. However, the definition of renal recovery is still heterogeneous across studies. This lack of a standardized definition for AKI and recovery has led to different values for the prevalence of renal recovery in the literature and, consequently, different assessments of CKD progression [7, 9, 18].

A main problem in defining recovery from AKI is the frequent absence of a baseline serum creatinine (SCr). Ideally, baseline creatinine should be considered as the last SCr measured in the previous 3–12 months. However, a significant proportion of patients have no previous assessment of SCr. In the absence of a baseline value, several approaches have been utilized to establish a baseline value [19], but these have been subject to over- or underestimation of AKI [20, 21]. While the hospital admission creatinine or the nadir during the event is often considered as representative of baseline renal function, these values are confounded by the factors leading to the admission, including hypotension, dehydration and nephrotoxin exposure. The best correlations with adjudicated cases have been observed for the mean outpatient creatinine values in the year prior to the event [20]. This standardization can improve the classification of patients and comparisons across studies, but depending on the population being studied, a higher proportion of patients with previous renal dysfunction would lead to underestimation of recovery. In addition, even patients showing complete recovery, as assessed based on SCr, can have loss of nephrons, as loss of more than half of function has to occur in order for SCr to be altered. This decrease in kidney functional reserve is one of the reasons why even complete recovery after an AKI episode can be associated with progression to CKD.

Another parameter that increases the inconsistency among studies is the time to assessing renal recovery. The timing of assessing renal recovery has been inconsistent across studies. Some studies have shown that recovery of renal function can continue after hospital discharge [22, 23]. Studies focusing on critically ill patients often follow patients for only a short time. In these studies, a significant proportion of patients die before renal recovery as a result of the underlying disease process or the complications associated with AKI. If renal recovery is evaluated while including all AKI patients, nonrenal recovery can be overestimated, as a proportion of patients who died could have had renal recovery if they had survived. The Acute Dialysis Quality Initiative definition standardizes the minimum follow-up period to 3 months to determine ESRD and helps to improve generalization across studies. Thus, studies should compare rates of recovery among standardized times, namely, at intensive care unit (ICU) or hospital discharge and at 90 days after discharge.

**Epidemiologic Data on Renal Recovery**

The prevalence of renal recovery varies depending on the studied population, the prevalence of CKD patients, and the definition of renal recovery. Bagshaw et al. [23] evaluated renal recovery in a cohort of 240 critically ill patients, including 45% with known CKD, who required dialysis. In total, 32% of survivors were on chronic renal replacement at hospital discharge. Schiffl et al. [24] followed 425 critically ill patients with acute tubular necrosis who required dialysis. At hospital discharge, 57% had normal renal function (SCr <1.3 mg/dl), 33% had SCr between 1.3 and 3 mg/dl, and 10% had SCr between 3 and 6 mg/dl. Metcalfe et al. [25], who included all hospitalized AKI patients, found an incidence of ESRD of 3% after 90 days among patients with previous normal renal function who required dialysis and an incidence of 16% among patients with previous renal dysfunction.

In a large population study from Scotland, Ali et al. [26] found an AKI incidence of 1,811 per million population and an incidence of acute-on-chronic renal failure of 336 per million population. The incidence of ESRD after 90 days was 0.6% in AKI patients. Full recovery, defined as creatinine above the threshold level for the RIFLE criteria, occurred in 92.5%, and partial recovery occurred in 7%. The incidence of ESRD was higher in patients with previous CKD; 6% were dialysis dependent after 90 days. In 2005, a multinational cohort study, which included more than 1,700 critically ill patients with severe but not only dialytic AKI across 23 countries, showed that 13.8% of survivors required dialysis at hospital discharge [27]. In a prospective study by Lins et al. [28], which included 293 patients with previous normal renal function and defined AKI as a creatinine above 2 mg/dl, 9.7% of survivors had a creatinine clearance below 15 ml/min at hospital discharge.

In a secondary analysis of the EPaNIC trial database, Schetz et al. [29], evaluated recovery of kidney function in patients who had developed AKI in the ICU by hospital discharge. Of the 1,310 AKI patients, 977 were discharged alive from the hospital, and rate of complete recovery (absence of KDIGO criteria) was markedly higher in survivors than in all AKI patients (79.5 vs. 67.0%), especially for more severe forms of AKI. When complete recovery was defined as a complete return to baseline sCr or as a return to below 1.25 times the baseline, the proportion of complete recovery in survivors decreased from 79.4 to 42 or 66%, respectively. These studies highlight the need for more comprehensive reporting of the populations being studied, the criteria used and the timing of assessment.

**Progression to Chronic Kidney Disease**

In studies including a long-term follow-up, the evidence suggests that recovery continues to occur after hospital discharge and peaks between 90 days and 6 months [23, 25, 30–33]. There are few recent studies that followed patients for longer periods of time [32–34]. Using data from the National Health and Nutrition Examination Surveys (NHANES), Hsu et al. [35] showed that the growth in incident ESRD overcame the growth in prevalent CKD, demonstrating that the rise of ESRD is not simply due to an increasing number of CKD patients. Using the Nationwide Inpatient Sample data, Waikar et al. [36] showed an increased incidence of AKI between 1988 and 2002, from 61 to 288 per 100,000 population, and an increase in survivors of dialysis-requiring acute renal failure, from 2.4 to 19.4 per 100,000 population. The annual incidence of ESRD among AKI survivors increased from 0.4 to 4.9 per 100,000 population between 1998 and 2002, while the overall incidence of ESRD in the USA increased from 16 to 34 per 100,000 population [36]. Several other studies in the last decade have supported the concept that AKI is a major risk factor for the development of CKD. Using a 5% random sample of Medicare beneficiaries in the USA, Ishani et al. found that in hospitalized patients older than 67 years, AKI was associated with a nearly sevenfold increase in the development of ESRD during the following 2 years, in comparison to patients who did not develop AKI [9]. The authors showed that when stratified on the basis of preexisting CKD, acute-on-chronic kidney disease was associated with a 41-fold increase in the development of ESRD; de novo AKI, with a 13-fold increase; and CKD in the absence of AKI, with a nearly 8.5-fold increase in comparison to patients without either acute or chronic kidney disease.

Using administrative databases from the Canadian province of Ontario, Wald et al. [37] found an incidence rate of ESRD of 26.3 per 1,000 person-years among 3,769 people who survived an episode of AKI requiring dialysis and were dialysis independent 30 days after hospital discharge, compared to an incidence of 9.1 per 1,000 person-years among 13,598 matched controls who did not have AKI, for an adjusted hazard ratio of 3.2. The authors did not observe an increase in long-term mortality risk associated with AKI. Lo et al. [8] evaluated the risk of progressive CKD in a cohort of 556,090 adult patients with baseline estimated glomerular filtration rates (GFRs) of at least 45 ml/min per 1.73 $m^2$ who were hospitalized in the Kaiser Permanente Northern California health system over an 8-year period. Patients who had dialysis-requiring AKI but were dialysis independent 30 days after hospital discharge had a 28-fold higher risk of having an estimated GFR less than 30 ml/min per 1.73 $m^2$ compared to patients who did not have dialysis-requiring AKI. Unlike the study by Wald et al., however, Lo et al. found a more than twofold increased risk of death in patients with AKI-requiring dialysis.

Bagshaw et al. evaluated the renal function of patients with severe AKI after 1 year of follow-up. The study showed that for patients who recovered, the renal function after 90 days was similar to the function after 1 year [23]. In a cohort of 79,000 in-patients at the Veterans Affairs Medical Center, Amdur et al. [2] evaluated the outcomes of 5,404 patients with a diagnosis of AKI based on International Classification of Diseases-9 codes. Patients were excluded from the study if they had preexisting CKD. The authors showed that patients with AKI were significantly more likely to progress to CKD over a 5-year follow-up period compared to a control group composed of in-patients with myocardial infarction or pneumonia and without AKI. Compared to the control group, AKI patients were at higher risk for progressing to CKD stage 4 and had a higher mortality rate.

**Determinants of Renal Recovery**

Which factors are associated with renal recovery after an episode of AKI is currently not clear. Many risk factors have been identified for the development of AKI, but their impact on renal recovery has only been evaluated in a minority of studies. The main risk factors influencing renal outcomes are advanced age and the presence of CKD, presumably due to the already decreasing renal function reserve observed in this population (fig. 1) [38].

Several studies have evaluated the effect of age on renal recovery. Macedo et al. [22] evaluated 84 survivors from an AKI episode who were followed by the same nephrologist for a median of 4.1 years. Renal recovery was defined as a GFR value higher than 60 ml/min per 1.73 $m^2$ and occurred in 19% at discharge and in 64%

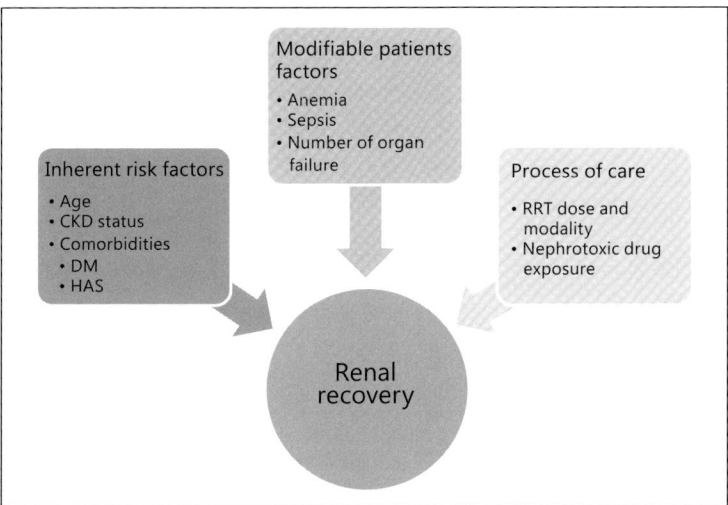

**Fig. 1.** Factors affecting renal recovery.

by 18 months. Age and SCr at hospital discharge were independent factors associated with nonrenal recovery, while AKI severity was not associated. Ishani et al. [9] found that patients older than 67 years old had a higher risk of ESRD among patients with previously decreased renal function. In a study by Pannu et al. [39], a lower baseline GFR pre-AKI was associated with more frequent ESRD and dialysis requirements post-hospital discharge. In an analysis by Hsu et al. [40], hospitalized patients who experienced AKI and CKD more frequently had ESRD within 1 month post-discharge compared to CKD patients without AKI. A recent meta-analysis by Coca et al. [5] demonstrated that AKI is an independent risk factor for CKD, ESRD and death. Nevertheless, not all studies have confirmed the association between CKD and lower renal recovery post-AKI. In a subanalysis of the Acute Renal Failure Trial Network (ATN) trial, Srisawat et al. could not show an association between baseline SCr and urine output at termination of dialysis and renal recovery. However, the trial excluded CKD stages 4 and 5 [38].

In addition to age and baseline renal function, presence of diabetes is a well-defined risk factor for AKI and CKD. Thakar et al. analyzed over 4,000 diabetics from a Veterans Affairs Medicare system and found that diabetic patients who were hospitalized for AKI had a significantly higher risk of progression to CKD stage 4 than patients who had not experienced any AKI did, regardless of the baseline GFR. A third of those patients hospitalized for AKI had subsequent repeated episodes of AKI, and each of these episodes had a cumulative dose-response association with the risk of reaching stage 4 CKD. The authors also showed that increased baseline SCr, hypertension and proteinuria were factors associated with CKD progression [41].

Renal recovery is also impaired by patients' general co-morbidity status. In a subset of patients from the ATN trial, the Charlson Comorbidity Index score was independently predictive of poor renal recovery. The association was increased when patient age was also considered [38]. Bucaloiu et al. retrospectively analyzed the influence of different factors on mortality and the development of CKD after recovery from AKI in a propensity score-matched cohort. They identified increasing age, the Charlson Comorbidity Index score, baseline hypoalbuminemia, congestive heart failure and hypertension to be associated with unfavorable outcomes [17]. In a cohort of 934 AKI patients, Lu et al. [42] found that the number of organ failures was an independent risk factor for nonrenal recovery. In a trial by Druml et al. [43], the mortality risk attributed to AKI seemed to be reduced in obese patients, but the relationship between obesity and renal recovery remains to be elucidated [44, 45].

**Potentially Modifiable Risk Factors Associated with Renal Recovery**

Although the knowledge of patient co-morbidities and their effect on renal recovery is fundamental in selecting patients for follow-up, few studies have focused on possible modifiable factors and their influence on renal recovery. Common in the CKD and elderly populations, anemia is a factor expected to be associated with decreased renal recovery. Few studies have evaluated the role of anemia in renal recovery from AKI. In an analysis of the Program to Improve Care in Acute Renal Disease (PICARD) cohort [46], composed of 32% CKD patients and with more than 50% of patients receiving dialysis, the authors were able to demonstrate an association between anemia and renal recovery. Renal recovery was significantly higher in patients with hemoglobin (Hb) higher 8 mg/dl, and renal recovery was 3 times more frequent in patients with a minimum Hb during the ICU stay higher than 9.5 mg/dl. In a cohort of 211 AKI patients in which 86% were considered anemic (Hb less than 9 or a decrease >2 mg/dl), Hu et al. [47] found that patients who recovered renal function had a greater decline in Hb and more often had acute anemia, advanced congenital hepatic fibrosis and a need for dialysis [47]. In contrast to the PICARD study, Hu et al. included all hospitalized patients, of whom only a third needed ICU admission and 8% needed dialysis, demonstrating that the effect of anemia is probably more pronounced in more severe cases of AKI, in which the effect of prolonged hypoxia could interfere with the degree and rate of renal recovery. Correction of anemia could help to restore renal oxygenation and perfusion pressure and decrease the time to renal recovery with different degrees of effectiveness, depending on the patient's other risk factors. Pre-operative anemia is highly prevalent, and several studies have shown that a management plan for the correction of anemia is fundamental to improve patient safety and outcome [48, 49].

Increasing severity of critical illness has been associated with poor renal recovery. In a trial by Mehta et al. [50], patients with an Acute Physiology, Age, Chronic Health Evaluation III score >100 experienced less renal recovery than those with a score of 81–100 or <79. Clinical prediction scores have also been described to predict renal recovery. Srisawat et al. [38] found a clinical model including age, SCr, pneumonia severity and nonrenal organ failure to be moderately predictive of renal recovery, defined as being alive and not being on dialysis or being classified as RIFLE-F by hospital discharge, with an AUC of 0.74.

**Process of Care**

It is increasingly accepted that fluid overload is associated with higher mortality. Heung et al. [51] have described a lower rate of renal recovery, defined as dependence in patients with fluid overload (>10% at RRT initiation), in a retrospective analysis of 170 hospitalized patients. Similar results were observed for the PICARD group, with a decreased likelihood of recovery in patients who experienced fluid overload at peak SCr [52]. Whether this is a reflection of the severity of disease or an independent risk factor remains to be proven, but it is plausible to believe that there is significant renal congestion associated with fluid overload, with or without abdominal compartment syndrome.

Procedures and medications may also influence renal prognosis. Acute respiratory distress syndrome, ventilator support and requirement of antibiotics have been associated with a negative impact on the recovery of renal function in a group of critically ill AKI patients requiring dialysis. These factors may represent a general assessment of the severity of critical disease, rather than independent risk factors for poor renal recovery, and need to be further evaluated. In contrast, nutritional support may offer positive renal effects. In a 2012 Cochrane Database Systematic Review, intravenous essential L-amino acids were associated with a significantly increased rate of recovery from AKI (risk ratio 1.70, 95% CI 1.70–2.79) and increased survival in dialyzed patients (risk ratio 3.56, 95% CI 0.97–13.08) compared to hypertonic glucose alone [53].

Early nephrology consultation for hospital-acquired AKI has been associated with a reduced need for RRT, reduced mortality and a reduced length of hospital stay. In a retrospective study by Meier et al., noncritically ill patients with no or late (>5 days) referral to nephrology for hospital-acquired AKI had lower rates of partial and complete recovery compared to early nephrology referral groups. The need for RRT during and after the hospital stay was significantly higher in patients with late versus early nephrology involvement [54]. This may be explained by the early identification of and intervention in modifiable patient risk factors, such as suspension of nephrotoxic medication or prevention of fluid overload. Additionally, follow-up of these patients is recommended at 3 months to evaluate new onset or worsening of CKD [55].

**Influence of Renal Replacement Therapy Dose and Modality on Renal Recovery**

The influence of dialysis dose and modality on the odds of renal recovery is another important issue. The Randomized Evaluation of Normal versus Augmented Level Renal Replacement Therapy (RENAL) and the ATN study [56, 57] are two recent multicenter trials that provided insights into the impact of RRT on renal recovery. These studies have shown that an improvement in patient survival or renal recovery could not be achieved by increasing the intensity of RRT. However, differences between these two trials provide data to argue that there may be an effect of the RRT modality on renal recovery. In the RENAL study, all 1,508 patients meeting the inclusion criteria received continuous RRT (CRRT) in the form of continuous venovenous hemodiafiltration. In the ATN study, of the 1,124 patients, those with cardiovascular stability were allocated to receive intermittent hemodialysis (IHD), and those with cardiovascular instability received CRRT in the form of continuous venovenous hemodiafiltration. Survivors in the RENAL study demonstrated a 13.3% rate of RRT dependence at day 28, compared to 45.2% in the ATN study. In the ATN study, at day 60, 24.6% of survivors remained RRT dependent, which was a higher rate than among RENAL survivors, of whom 5.6% were RRT dependent at day 90. In addition, in the ATN trial, the mean number of RRT-free days at 28 days was 6.5, and in the RENAL trial, it was 17. In the ATN trial, 37% of the IHD sessions were complicated by hypotension, which could explain the delayed renal recovery associated with IHD. CRRT could be associated with fewer episodes of hypotension and may offer better control over fluid balance. Other recent studies from observational cohorts have also suggested a recovery benefit for CRRT in comparison to intermittent techniques [58].

**Conclusion**

Recovery from AKI is a potentially modifiable event and should be targeted by therapy. Some factors associated with lower rates of recovery are nonmodifiable, such as advanced age, diabetes, preexisting CKD and the overall co-morbid burden.

Efforts should be made to identify the possible clinical and therapeutic factors in which we may intervene to positively influence renal outcomes, such as prevention of hypotension and anemia, avoidance of fluid overload, scheduling of prompt nephrology consultation for AKI, and prevention of subsequent episodes of AKI. Outpatient renal follow-up is fundamental for those patients with previous CKD and for those who have not recovered from an AKI episode, as they are at increased risk for progression to ESRD. Renal recovery must be evaluated within 3 months to 1 year after an AKI episode. Nephrology referral should be considered for older patients and those with elevated SCr at hospital discharge. These practices will help to stop the growing incidence of ESRD derived from AKI episodes.

## References

1 Chawla LS, Amdur RL, Amodeo S, Kimmel PL, Palant CE: The severity of acute kidney injury predicts progression to chronic kidney disease. Kidney Int 2011;79:1361–1369.
2 Amdur RL, Chawla LS, Amodeo S, Kimmel PL, Palant CE: Outcomes following diagnosis of acute renal failure in U.S. veterans: focus on acute tubular necrosis. Kidney Int 2009; 76:1089–1097.
3 Bagshaw SM, George C, Bellomo R, Committe ADM: A comparison of the RIFLE and AKIN criteria for acute kidney injury in critically ill patients. Nephrol Dial Transplant 2008;23:1569–1574.
4 Ali T, Khan I, Simpson W, Prescott G, Townend J, Smith W, et al: Incidence and outcomes in acute kidney injury: a comprehensive population-based study. J Am Soc Nephrol 2007;18:1292–1298.
5 Coca SG, Singanamala S, Parikh CR: Chronic kidney disease after acute kidney injury: a systematic review and meta-analysis. Kidney Int 2012;81:442–448.
6 Chawla LS, Kimmel PL: Acute kidney injury and chronic kidney disease: an integrated clinical syndrome. Kidney Int 2012;82:516–524.
7 Wald R, Quinn RR, Luo J, Li P, Scales DC, Mamdani MM, et al: Chronic dialysis and death among survivors of acute kidney injury requiring dialysis. JAMA 2009;302:1179–1185.
8 Lo LJ, Go AS, Chertow GM, McCulloch CE, Fan D, Ordonez JD, et al: Dialysis-requiring acute renal failure increases the risk of progressive chronic kidney disease. Kidney Int 2009;76:893–899.
9 Ishani A, Xue JL, Himmelfarb J, Eggers PW, Kimmel PL, Molitoris BA, et al: Acute kidney injury increases risk of ESRD among elderly. J Am Soc Nephrol 2009;20:223–228.
10 Lafrance JP, Miller DR: Acute kidney injury associates with increased long-term mortality. J Am Soc Nephrol 2010;21:345–352.
11 Bhandari S, Turney JH: Survivors of acute renal failure who do not recover renal function. QJM 1996;89:415–421.
12 Schiffl H: Renal recovery from acute tubular necrosis requiring renal replacement therapy: a prospective study in critically ill patients. Nephrol Dial Transplant 2006;21:1248–1252.
13 Ponte B, Tenorio MT, Hiller R, Candela A, Liaño F: Continuous dialysis by gravity through the filter of the extracorporeal membrane oxygenation. Nephrol Dial Transplant 2007;22:3676–3677.
14 Liu KD, Lo L, Hsu CY: Some methodological issues in studying the long-term renal sequelae of acute kidney injury. Curr Opin Nephrol Hypertens 2009;18:241–245.
15 Ishani A, Xue JL, Himmelfarb J, Eggers PW, Kimmel PL, Molitoris BA, et al: Acute kidney injury increases risk of ESRD among elderly. J Am Soc Nephrol. 2009;20:223–228.
16 Jones J, Holmen J, De Graauw J, Jovanovich A, Thornton S, Chonchol M: Association of complete recovery from acute kidney injury with incident CKD stage 3 and all-cause mortality. Am J Kidney Dis 2012;60:402–408.

17 Bucaloiu ID, Kirchner HL, Norfolk ER, Hartle JE 2nd, Perkins RM: Increased risk of death and de novo chronic kidney disease following reversible acute kidney injury. Kidney Int 2012;81:477–485.

18 Coca SG, Yusuf B, Shlipak MG, Garg AX, Parikh CR: Long-term risk of mortality and other adverse outcomes after acute kidney injury: a systematic review and meta-analysis. Am J Kidney Dis 2009;53:961–973.

19 Siew ED, Matheny ME, Ikizler TA, Lewis JB, Miller RA, Waitman LR, et al: Commonly used surrogates for baseline renal function affect the classification and prognosis of acute kidney injury. Kidney Int 2010;77:536–542.

20 Siew ED, Ikizler TA, Matheny ME, Shi Y, Schildcrout JS, Danciu I, et al: Estimating baseline kidney function in hospitalized patients with impaired kidney function. Clin J Am Soc Nephrol 2012;7:712–719.

21 Siew ED, Peterson JF, Eden SK, Moons KG, Ikizler TA, Matheny ME: Use of multiple imputation method to improve estimation of missing baseline serum creatinine in acute kidney injury research. Clin J Am Soc Nephrol 2013;8:10–18.

22 Macedo E, Zanetta DMT, Abdulkader RCRM: Long-term follow-up of patients after acute kidney injury: patterns of renal functional recovery. Plos One 2012;7:e36388.

23 Bagshaw SM, Laupland KB, Doig CJ, Mortis G, Fick GH, Mucenski M, et al: Prognosis for long-term survival and renal recovery in critically ill patients with severe acute renal failure: a population-based study. Crit Care 2005;9:R700–R709.

24 Schiffl H: Renal recovery from acute tubular necrosis requiring renal replacement therapy: a prospective study in critically ill patients. Nephrol Dial Transplant 2006;21:1248–1252.

25 Metcalfe W, Simpson M, Khan IH, Prescott GJ, Simpson K, Smith WC, et al: Acute renal failure requiring renal replacement therapy: incidence and outcome. QJM 2002;95:579–583.

26 Ali T, Khan I, Simpson W, Prescott G, Townend J, Smith W, et al: Incidence and outcomes in acute kidney injury: a comprehensive population-based study. J Am Soc Nephrol 2007;18:1292–1298.

27 Uchino S, Kellum JA, Bellomo R, Doig GS, Morimatsu H, Morgera S, et al: Acute renal failure in critically ill patients: a multinational, multicenter study. JAMA 2005;294:813–818.

28 Lins RL, Elseviers MM, Daelemans R: Severity scoring and mortality 1 year after acute renal failure. Nephrol Dial Transplant 2006;21:1066–1068.

29 Schetz M, Gunst J, De Vlieger G, Van den Berghe G: Recovery from AKI in the critically ill: potential confounders in the evaluation. Intensive Care Med 2015;41:1648–1657.

30 Kjellstrand CM, Ebben J, Davin T: Time of death, recovery of renal function, development of chronic renal failure and need for chronic hemodialysis in patients with acute tubular necrosis. Trans Am Soc Artif Intern Organs 1981;27:45–50.

31 Hall JW, Johnson WJ, Maher FT, Hunt JC: Immediate and long-term prognosis in acute renal failure. Ann Intern Med 1970;73:515–521.

32 Liano F, Felipe C, Tenorio MT, Rivera M, Abraira V, Saez-de-Urturi JM, et al: Long-term outcome of acute tubular necrosis: a contribution to its natural history. Kidney Int 2007;71:679–686.

33 Bell M, Granath F, Schon S, Ekbom A, Martling CR: Continuous renal replacement therapy is associated with less chronic renal failure than intermittent haemodialysis after acute renal failure. Intensive Care Med 2007;33:773–780.

34 Morgera S, Kraft AK, Siebert G, Luft FC, Neumayer HH: Long-term outcomes in acute renal failure patients treated with continuous renal replacement therapies. Am J Kidney Dis 2002;40:275–279.

35 Hsu CY, Vittinghoff E, Lin F, Shlipak MG: The incidence of end-stage renal disease is increasing faster than the prevalence of chronic renal insufficiency. Ann Intern Med 2004;141:95–101.

36 Waikar SS, Curhan GC, Wald R, McCarthy EP, Chertow GM: Declining mortality in patients with acute renal failure, 1988 to 2002. J Am Soc Nephrol 2006;17:1143–1150.

37 Wald R, Quinn RR, Luo J, Li P, Scales DC, Mamdani MM, et al: Chronic dialysis and death among survivors of acute kidney injury requiring dialysis. JAMA 2009;302:1179–1185.

38 Srisawat N, Wen X, Lee M, Kong L, Elder M, Carter M, et al: Urinary biomarkers and renal recovery in critically ill patients with renal support. Clin J Am Soc Nephrol 2011;6:1815–1823.

39 Pannu N, James M, Hemmelgarn BR, Dong J, Tonelli M, Klarenbach S, et al: Modification of outcomes after acute kidney injury by the presence of CKD. Am J Kidney Dis 2011;58: 206–213.

40 Hsu CY, Chertow GM, McCulloch CE, Fan D, Ordonez JD, Go AS: Nonrecovery of kidney function and death after acute on chronic renal failure. Clin J Am Soc Nephrol 2009;4: 891–898.

41 Thakar CV, Christianson A, Himmelfarb J, Leonard AC: Acute kidney injury episodes and chronic kidney disease risk in diabetes mellitus. Clin J Am Soc Nephrol 2011;6:2567–2572.

42 Lu R, Muciño-Bermejo MJ, Armignacco P, Fang Y, Cai H, Zhang M, et al: Survey of acute kidney injury and related risk factors of mortality in hospitalized patients in a third-level urban hospital of Shanghai. Blood Purif 2014;38:140–148.

43 Druml W, Metnitz B, Schaden E, Bauer P, Metnitz PG: Impact of body mass on incidence and prognosis of acute kidney injury requiring renal replacement therapy. Intensive Care Med 2010;36:1221–1228.

44 Shashaty MG, Meyer NJ, Localio AR, Gallop R, Bellamy SL, Holena DN, et al: African American race, obesity, and blood product transfusion are risk factors for acute kidney injury in critically ill trauma patients. J Crit Care 2012;27:496–504.

45 Myrvang H: Acute kidney injury: obesity is associated with AKI after surgery via oxidative stress. Nat Rev Nephrol 2012;8:433.

46 Macedo E, Bouchard J, Chertow GM, Himmelfarb J, Ikizler TA, Mehta RL: Severity of anemia is associated with AKI recovery during ICU stay. Kidney Week 2014, Philadelphia, 2014.

47 Hu SL, Said FR, Epstein D, Lokeshwari M: The impact of anemia on renal recovery and survival in acute kidney injury. Clin Nephrol 2013;79:221–228.

48 Shema-Didi L, Ore L, Geron R, Kristal B: Is anemia at hospital admission associated with in-hospital acute kidney injury occurrence? Nephron Clin Pract 2010;115:c168–c176.

49 Kim CJ, Connell H, McGeorge AD, Hu R: Prevalence of preoperative anaemia in patients having first-time cardiac surgery and its impact on clinical outcome. A retrospective observational study. Perfusion 2015;30:277–283.

50 Mehta RL, McDonald B, Gabbai FB, Pahl M, Pascual MT, Farkas A, et al: A randomized clinical trial of continuous versus intermittent dialysis for acute renal failure. Kidney Int 2001;60:1154–1163.

51 Heung M, Wolfgram DF, Kommareddi M, Hu Y, Song PX, Ojo AO: Fluid overload at initiation of renal replacement therapy is associated with lack of renal recovery in patients with acute kidney injury. Nephrol Dial Transplant 2012;27:956–961.

52 Bouchard J, Soroko SB, Chertow GM, Himmelfarb J, Ikizler TA, Paganini EP, et al: Fluid accumulation, survival and recovery of kidney function in critically ill patients with acute kidney injury. Kidney Int 2009;76:422–427.

53 Li Y, Tang X, Zhang J, Wu T: Nutritional support for acute kidney injury. The Cochrane Database Syst Rev 2012;8:CD005426.

54 Meier P, Bonfils RM, Vogt B, Burnand B, Burnier M: Referral patterns and outcomes in noncritically ill patients with hospital-acquired acute kidney injury. Clin J Am Soc Nephrol 2011;6:2215–2225.

55 Khwaja A: KDIGO clinical practice guidelines for acute kidney injury. Nephron Clin Pract 2012;120:179–184.

56 Bellomo R, Cass A, Cole L, Finfer S, Gallagher M, Lo S, et al: Intensity of continuous renal-replacement therapy in critically ill patients. N Engl J Med 2009;361:1627–1638.

57 Palevsky PM, Zhang JH, O'Connor TZ, Chertow GM, Crowley ST, Choudhury D, et al: Intensity of renal support in critically ill patients with acute kidney injury. N Engl J Med 2008;359:7–20.

58 Wald R, Shariff SZ, Adhikari NK, Bagshaw SM, Burns KE, Friedrich JO, et al: The association between renal replacement therapy modality and long-term outcomes among critically ill adults with acute kidney injury: a retrospective cohort study*. Crit Care Med 2014;42:868–877.

Ravindra L. Mehta, MD
Division of Nephrology and Hypertension
Department of Medicine, University of California San Diego
200 W Arbor Drive, Mail Code 8342
San Diego, CA 92103 (USA)
E-Mail rmehta@ucsd.edu

# Pathophysiology of Septic Acute Kidney Injury

Johan Mårtensson[a, b] · Rinaldo Bellomo[a, c]

[a]Department of Intensive Care, Austin Hospital, Melbourne, Vic., Australia; [b]Section of Anaesthesia and Intensive Care Medicine, Department of Physiology and Pharmacology, Karolinska Institutet, Stockholm, Sweden; [c]Australian and New Zealand Intensive Care Research Centre (ANZIC-RC), Department of Epidemiology and Preventive Medicine, Monash University, Melbourne, Vic., Australia

## Abstract

**Background:** Despite increased understanding of the pathophysiology of septic acute kidney injury (AKI), treatment options are limited, and mortality remains high. **Summary:** Septic AKI is triggered by pathogen-associated molecular patterns from bacteria and damage-associated molecular patterns released from or exposed on damaged cells. Downstream effects include glomerular and peritubular endothelial dysfunction, downregulation of tubular reabsorptive work, cell-cycle arrest, regulated cell death and destruction of damaged cell organelles. In the laboratory, pharmacological modulation of some of these pathways prevents AKI or enhances recovery from AKI, yet no data exist to support the utility of such AKI therapy in man. However, avoiding systemic and renal venous congestion, hypotension and fluid overload attenuates AKI in critically ill septic patients. **Key Message:** While therapies aiming at modulating the sepsis-induced cellular response are discovered and tested, hemodynamic optimization remains critical in patients with or at risk of AKI.

© 2016 S. Karger AG, Basel

Sepsis is the major trigger of acute kidney injury (AKI) in critically ill patients [1]. In severe cases, such sepsis-induced AKI is associated with mortality rates above 50% [2]. Furthermore, survivors carry a several-fold increased risk of chronic renal impairment [3].

Sepsis is caused by the innate immune system's response to invading microbes. This vital immune response attacks foreign pathogens, attenuating their proliferation and spread in the affected tissue. However, activated circulating immune mediators also pose an immediate threat to native cells distant from the site of infection. The kidney parenchyma is particularly exposed to such mediators since it receives and filters a large proportion of toxin-rich blood delivered by cardiac output.

The pathophysiological events leading to AKI and the timing of such events during its development are not completely understood. However, several important cellular responses have been observed in animal models of septic AKI. These responses are important since they provide plausible explanations of the connection between cellular injury and functional deterioration and because some of these cellular responses can be pharmacologically modified and therefore provide targets for future therapies.

In this chapter, we discuss three topical cellular mechanisms involved in septic AKI: cellular activation, hibernation, and suicide. Moreover, the connection between cellular injury and kidney dysfunction is reviewed. Finally, we describe the role of systemic and renal hemodynamics in septic AKI.

## Cellular Activation

Invading bacteria release a variety of so-called pathogen-associated molecular patterns (PAMPs), which activate the innate immune response by binding pattern recognition receptors on immune cells. In addition, numerous native molecules, collectively called damage-associated molecular patterns (DAMPs), are released by damaged cells at the site of infection, interact with pattern recognition receptors, and further amplify the systemic inflammatory response (fig. 1) [4].

In addition to their ability to activate immune cells, PAMPs and DAMPs bind to and activate many other cell types, including kidney endothelial, glomerular and tubular cells. Endothelial cell activation causes important structural changes in the glomerular and peritubular capillaries. The expression of adhesion molecules facilitates binding of neutrophils and platelets to the endothelial surface and activates these cells to release coagulation factors and inflammatory mediators [5]. Consequently, inflammation is triggered and maintained in tissues such as the kidneys, distant from the primary site of infection.

Proteolytic enzymes and reactive oxygen species (ROS) released from immune cells contribute to tissue breakdown. In particular, breakdown of endothelial glycocalyx, tight junctions between cells and basement membrane collagen impairs vascular stability, causing vascular leakage and interstitial edema [6, 7], with extended injury to the kidney parenchyma.

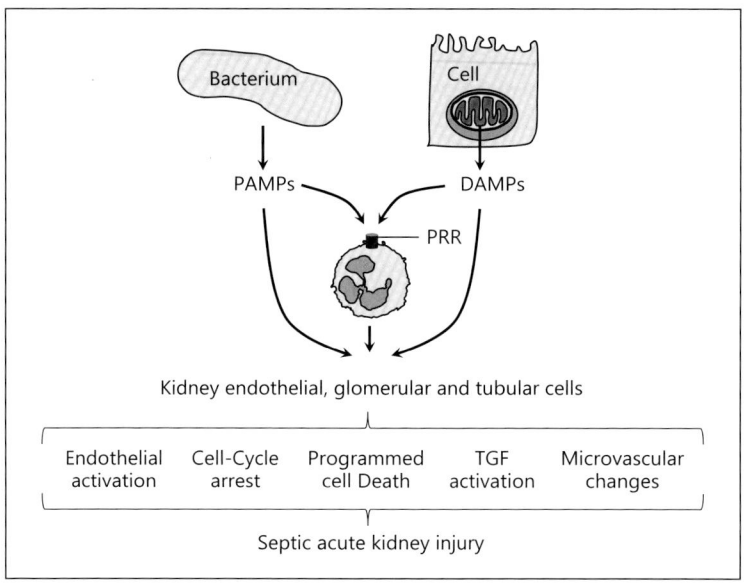

**Fig. 1.** Pathophysiology of septic acute kidney injury. PAMPs = Pathogen-associated molecular patterns; DAMPs = damage-associated molecular patterns; PRR = pattern recognition receptors; TGF = tubuloglomerular feedback.

Similarly, tubular epithelial cells are activated by PAMPs and DAMPs from the glomerular filtrate as well as from the surrounding peritubular circulation. In response to this toxic environment, upregulated synthesis and release of apparently protective proteins are seen. Neutrophil gelatinase-associated lipocalin (NGAL) and hepcidin are two such proteins and are critically involved in controlling iron balance and indirectly regulating ROS generation [8]. Free iron catalyzes the extracellular conversion to ROS and may therefore contribute to cell membrane damage during systemic inflammation. In addition, intracellular iron-dependent lipid peroxidation and necrosis (known as ferroptosis) appears to be an important mechanism during postischemic and toxic AKI [9].

Tubular NGAL synthesis and release into the bloodstream and urine are upregulated during inflammation and oxidative stress [10]. Via its ability to bind iron-binding molecules (siderophores), NGAL captures extracellular iron and facilitates intracellular iron delivery and storage. In addition to NGAL, hepcidin synthesis is induced during cellular stress [8]. Hepcidin binds to and degrades ferroportin, an iron exporter located in the outer cell membrane of tubular cells. Together with NGAL, hepcidin thereby contributes to sequestration of intracellular iron, which in turn mitigates extracellular iron-induced cell damage. NGAL's renoprotective role was demonstrated in animal models of ischemia-reperfusion-induced AKI. In those studies, rapid uptake of intravenously infused NGAL by proximal tubular cells was found to improve cell proliferation and attenuate tubular damage and apoptosis [11, 12].

**Cellular Hibernation**

Logically, a cell's response to stressors such as inflammatory mediators would be to stop its energy-consuming activities. Indeed, several studies have provided evidence that such 'cellular hibernation' may actually occur. Approximately 80% of renal oxygen consumption is used by the $Na^+$-$K^+$ ATPase for reabsorption of sodium [13]. Relocation of the tubular sodium pumps from the basolateral to the apical or lateral membrane, as seen during inflammation [14], effectively stops their machinery, causing a significant reduction in oxygen consumption. Moreover, receptors responsible for proximal tubular reabsorption of proteins, e.g. the megalin receptor, are downregulated, further reducing cellular energy demands [15]. Another important aspect is the fact that such megalin receptor downregulation prevents reabsorption and intracellular accumulation of filtered inflammatory toxins, thereby protecting tubular cells against further injury.

It is well known that the kidney can recover from insults exerted by nephrotoxins, ischemia-reperfusion injury and sepsis. Renal recovery depends on the ability of surviving tubular cells to proliferate to replace damaged cells [16]. However, some tubular cells enter proliferative cell-cycle arrest in response to stress. This experimental observation is supported by human data showing elevated urinary levels of proteins responsible for cell-cycle inhibition in critically ill patients [17]. Furthermore, cell-cycle arrest appears to contribute to the initiation of AKI during sepsis in rats [18], and higher urinary cell-cycle arrest biomarker levels were observed in patients with severe AKI compared to non-AKI controls in some studies [19, 20]. Finally, although cell-cycle arrest may be an important protective mechanism during cellular insults – reduced oxygen consumption and the prevention of mitosis in damaged cells will protect an organ from extended injuries – restarting the cell cycle once the insult has abated appears important for renal recovery [18].

**Cellular Suicide**

The cell's ability to commit suicide is a major protective process during intracellular infections. However, such regulated cell death is also triggered when PAMPs and DAMPs, released during sepsis, bind to cell-surface receptors. In the setting of sepsis, cell death may therefore accelerate inflammation and tissue injury.

Apoptosis is one form of regulated cell death consistently observed in experimental and human AKI [21, 22]. This caspase-dependent process involves cell fragmentation into apoptotic bodies that are phagocytosed, degraded and effectively removed without release of intracellular contents.

Necroptosis, another form of programmed cell death triggered by the interaction and activation of receptor-interacting protein kinase (RIPK) 1 and 3, is characterized by plasma membrane rupture and release of intracellular contents, including DAMPs, into the circulation. Consequently, necroptosis is a more potent inflammatory accelerator than apoptosis is, and drugs blocking the necroptotic pathways are currently being explored. In fact, whereas blocking of apoptotic pathways failed to improve survival during tumor necrosis factor-alpha- or sepsis-induced systemic inflammation in mice, deletion of RIPK3 or pretreatment with an RIPK1 inhibitor (necrostatin-1) provided complete protection [23].

The functional importance of necroptosis and the renoprotective effect of necrostatin-1 in toxic and ischemia-reperfusion-related AKI has been demonstrated (table 1) [24, 25]. Whether this promising therapy is equally effective in preventing and treating sepsis-induced AKI is yet to be shown.

Mitochondrial damage is observed in severe sepsis [26]. In particular, mitochondrial membrane permeability changes, mitochondrial swelling and even rupture are seen in kidney tubules during experimental sepsis. Consequently, mitochondrial contents such as ROS and pro-apoptotic factors are released into the cell cytoplasm, damaging intracellular structures and causing oxidative stress and cell death. However, important intracellular processes are simultaneously induced to prevent cellular self-destruction. Autophagy is one such process by which damaged organelles, including mitochondria (then referred to as mitophagy), and toxins are sequestered within so-called autophagosomes that are subsequently delivered to lysosomes for degradation. It has therefore been suggested that autophagy plays an important cytoprotective role during septic AKI and that exhausted autophagy/mitophagy leads to progressive renal injury [27]. As molecular mechanisms are being untangled, autophagy may become a target for future AKI therapies. In addition, the potent immunosuppressant cyclosporine A, which interferes with mitochondrial stability, appears to protect against experimental AKI [28], although its utility in septic AKI is still unexplored (table 1).

**Connection between Tubular Injury and Impaired Glomerular Filtration**

Most studies exploring AKI pathogenesis have focused on tubular cell injury, whereas few have assessed the pathophysiology of the glomerulus. However, the most important clinical feature of AKI is an impaired glomerular filtration rate

**Table 1.** Potential therapeutic targets in septic AKI

| Mechanism | Role in AKI | Potential treatment |
|---|---|---|
| Apoptosis | Caspase-dependent cell death | Caspase inhibitors |
| Ferroptosis | Iron-dependent necrosis of tubular cells | Ferroptosis inhibitor (ferrostatin 16–86) |
| Necroptosis | RIPK1- and RIPK3-mediated necrosis of tubular cells | Necrostatin-1<br>Necrosulfonamide<br>RIPK3 inhibitors<br>Death-receptor antagonists<br>Plasma membrane channel blockers |
| Glycocalyx breakdown | Altered vascular permeability | Corticosteroids?<br>Antithrombin?<br>N-acetylcysteine? |
| Extracellular histones | DAMPs released by necroptotic cells | Anti-histone antibodies |
| VEGF | Binding to VEGFR2 increases vascular permeability | Anti-VEGF antibodies |
| Mitochondrial permeability transition | Release of ROS and pro-apoptotic factors, causing tubular cell injury/death | Cyclosporine A |

RIPK = Receptor-interacting protein kinase; DAMP = damage-associated molecular patterns; VEGF = vascular endothelial growth factor; VEGFR2 = vascular endothelial growth factor receptor 2; ROS = reactive oxygen species.

(GFR). It is possible that sepsis-induced alterations in the structure and function of the glomerular filtration barrier are disconnected from tubular injuries and independently explain the altered GFR. For example, specialized smooth-muscle cells, or so-called mesangial cells, lining the glomerular filter contract in response to inflammatory stimuli [29]. Contraction of the renal mesangium will logically reduce the glomerular pore size and reduce the GFR. The impact of this potential mechanism in septic AKI is, however, unknown.

Tubuloglomerular feedback activation may explain the link between tubular injury and the impaired GFR in sepsis. Since sodium reabsorption is impaired in the injured proximal tubule (see the 'Cellular Hibernation' section above), the 'salt-detecting' macula densa cells in the distal tubule are exposed to a higher sodium concentration. Consequently, sodium-induced activation of these salt detectors will trigger contraction of the afferent arteriole, thereby lowering the glomerular filtration pressure and GFR [30]. In fact, such an imbalance in the vasomotor tone of the afferent and efferent arterioles might explain the sometimes-dramatic decline in the GFR in the setting of increased renal blood flow (RBF) [31]. Finally, as will be discussed below, management of systemic hemodynamics in septic patients may have additional impact on kidney function.

**Renal Hemodynamics in Septic Acute Kidney Injury**

Renal hemodynamics are altered in patients with septic AKI. The contribution of these alterations to the initiation and maintenance of AKI is, however, uncertain. In addition, multiple interventions aiming to optimize cardiovascular function during sepsis may significantly modulate the AKI risk as well as the chance of renal recovery in patients with established AKI.

With the exception of patients with sepsis-induced myocardial stunning, high cardiac output, systemic vasodilation and hypotension are typically seen in patients with early septic shock. Simultaneously, renal vasodilation and increased RBF are observed in septic animals [31] as well as in patients [32]. In contrast, in septic patients with established AKI, reduced renal blood has been demonstrated using cine phase-contrast magnetic resonance imaging [33]. Collectively, these observations suggest that changes in the renal macrocirculation insufficiently explain deteriorating kidney dysfunction during septic AKI. However, novel techniques have revealed important alterations in the renal microcirculation during sepsis. Such alterations include convective oxygen shunting and reduction of capillary density, causing changes in the blood flow distribution, with areas of insufficient flow and ischemia [34].

Avoiding systemic hypotension is a cornerstone of the management of patients with or at risk of AKI. Optimal individual blood pressure targets are, however, difficult to predict. Observational data in patients with septic shock failed to demonstrate an independent association between mean arterial pressure (MAP) or MAP deficit (the difference between premorbid MAP and MAP in the intensive care unit) and worsening kidney function after controlling for other hemodynamic measures [35].

In contrast, more patients with chronic hypertension and septic shock developed severe AKI, requiring renal replacement therapy if their MAP was maintained at 65–70 mm Hg instead of 80–85 mm Hg, in a large randomized controlled trial [36]. Physiologically, 'sufficient' MAP is required to maintain the RBF and glomerular hydraulic pressure needed to maintain the GFR. Furthermore, sluggish RBF amplifies the harmful effects of circulating inflammatory toxins on kidney cells [34]. Based on the above-mentioned experimental and clinical observations, defining individual MAP targets should continue to be a priority in the care of septic patients and an aim of future trials.

Administration of intravenous fluids is commonly used to treat or prevent hypotension in septic patients. Unfortunately, fluid-induced AKI is a serious complication of such therapy [30]. Intravenous fluid administration improves MAP, RBF and the GFR in hypovolemic patients. In contrast, the effect on these parameters is either absent or transient in septic patients with vasoplegia and increased capillary leakiness [37, 38]. In such patients, excessive fluid administration may lead to renal interstitial edema, causing renal parenchymal hypertension with increased intratubular and renal venous pressures [39]. Raised intratubular pressure counteracts the GFR, whereas renal venous congestion lowers the transrenal pressure gradient (renal artery pressure – renal vein pressure) required to maintain RBF and the GFR.

In addition, especially in patients with impaired diastolic cardiac dysfunction or right heart failure, overzealous fluid administration will increase central venous pressure, further augmenting renal vein pressure and impairing RBF and the GFR. The renal consequences of fluid overload and venous congestion have been shown in several studies. The first studies found independent associations of fluid accumulation with AKI development [40] and progression and mortality [41, 42]. In addition, subsequent studies have confirmed that AKI progression is more strongly associated with elevated central venous pressure than with other hemodynamic indices, such as MAP, the cardiac index or pulmonary artery pressures [35, 43–45].

## Summary

The pathophysiology of septic AKI is complex. It includes adaptive cellular mechanisms, increased synthesis of iron scavengers to reduce ROS formation, reduced oxygen utilization, and self-destruction of injured cell organelles and entire cells. While these mechanisms appear initially protective, their prolonged activation may amplify the systemic inflammatory response, causing permanent kidney injuries. Novel therapies modulating these pathways are currently under intense investigation. In addition, prevention of venous congestion, hypotension and fluid overload may reduce AKI incidence in septic patients.

## References

1 Uchino S, Kellum JA, Bellomo R, Doig GS, Morimatsu H, Morgera S, Schetz M, Tan I, Bouman C, Macedo E, et al: Acute renal failure in critically ill patients: a multinational, multicenter study. JAMA 2005;294:813–818.
2 Bagshaw SM, Uchino S, Bellomo R, Morimatsu H, Morgera S, Schetz M, Tan I, Bouman C, Macedo E, Gibney N, et al: Septic acute kidney injury in critically ill patients: clinical characteristics and outcomes. Clin J Am Soc Nephrol 2007;2:431–439.
3 Rimes-Stigare C, Frumento P, Bottai M, Martensson J, Martling CR, Walther SM, Karlstrom G, Bell M: Evolution of chronic renal impairment and long-term mortality after de novo acute kidney injury in the critically ill; a Swedish multi-centre cohort study. Crit Care 2015;19:221.
4 Zhang Q, Raoof M, Chen Y, Sumi Y, Sursal T, Junger W, Brohi K, Itagaki K, Hauser CJ: Circulating mitochondrial DAMPs cause inflammatory responses to injury. Nature 2010; 464:104–107.
5 Verma SK, Molitoris BA: Renal endothelial injury and microvascular dysfunction in acute kidney injury. Semin Nephrol 2015;35: 96–107.
6 Tanaka T, Nangaku M: Angiogenesis and hypoxia in the kidney. Nat Rev Nephrol 2013; 9:211–222.
7 Chelazzi C, Villa G, Mancinelli P, De Gaudio AR, Adembri C: Glycocalyx and sepsis-induced alterations in vascular permeability. Crit Care 2015;19:26.
8 Martensson J, Glassford NJ, Jones S, Eastwood GM, Young H, Peck L, Ostland V, Westerman M, Venge P, Bellomo R: Urinary neutrophil gelatinase-associated lipocalin to hepcidin ratio as a biomarker of acute kidney injury in intensive care unit patients. Minerva Anestesiol 2015;81:1192–1200.
9 Linkermann A, Skouta R, Himmerkus N, Mulay SR, Dewitz C, De Zen F, Prokai A, Zuchtriegel G, Krombach F, Welz PS, et al: Synchronized renal tubular cell death involves ferroptosis. Proc Natl Acad Sci U S A 2014;111:16836–16841.
10 Martensson J, Bell M, Oldner A, Xu S, Venge P, Martling CR: Neutrophil gelatinase-associated lipocalin in adult septic patients with and without acute kidney injury. Intensive Care Med 2010;36:1333–1340.
11 Mori K, Lee HT, Rapoport D, Drexler IR, Foster K, Yang J, Schmidt-Ott KM, Chen X, Li JY, Weiss S, et al: Endocytic delivery of lipocalin-siderophore-iron complex rescues the kidney from ischemia-reperfusion injury. J Clin Invest 2005;115:610–621.
12 Mishra J, Mori K, Ma Q, Kelly C, Yang J, Mitsnefes M, Barasch J, Devarajan P: Amelioration of ischemic acute renal injury by neutrophil gelatinase-associated lipocalin. J Am Soc Nephrol 2004;15:3073–3082.
13 Ricksten SE, Bragadottir G, Redfors B: Renal oxygenation in clinical acute kidney injury. Crit Care 2013;17:221.
14 Zuk A, Bonventre JV, Brown D, Matlin KS: Polarity, integrin, and extracellular matrix dynamics in the postischemic rat kidney. Am J Physiol 1998;275:C711–C731.
15 Mahadevappa R, Nielsen R, Christensen EI, Birn H: Megalin in acute kidney injury: foe and friend. Am J Physiol Renal Physiol 2014; 306:F147–F154.
16 Humphreys BD, Valerius MT, Kobayashi A, Mugford JW, Soeung S, Duffield JS, McMahon AP, Bonventre JV: Intrinsic epithelial cells repair the kidney after injury. Cell Stem Cell 2008;2:284–291.
17 Bell M, Larsson A, Venge P, Bellomo R, Martensson J: Assessment of cell-cycle arrest biomarkers to predict early and delayed acute kidney injury. Dis Markers 2015;2015: 158658.
18 Yang QH, Liu DW, Long Y, Liu HZ, Chai WZ, Wang XT: Acute renal failure during sepsis: potential role of cell cycle regulation. J Infect 2009;58:459–464.
19 Kashani K, Al-Khafaji A, Ardiles T, Artigas A, Bagshaw SM, Bell M, Bihorac A, Birkhahn R, Cely CM, Chawla LS, et al: Discovery and validation of cell cycle arrest biomarkers in human acute kidney injury. Crit Care 2013; 17:R25.
20 Bihorac A, Chawla LS, Shaw AD, Al-Khafaji A, Davison DL, Demuth GE, Fitzgerald R, Gong MN, Graham DD, Gunnerson K, et al: Validation of cell-cycle arrest biomarkers for acute kidney injury using clinical adjudication. Am J Respir Crit Care Med 2014;189: 932–939.
21 Havasi A, Borkan SC: Apoptosis and acute kidney injury. Kidney Int 2011;80:29–40.

22 Lerolle N, Nochy D, Guerot E, Bruneval P, Fagon JY, Diehl JL, Hill G: Histopathology of septic shock induced acute kidney injury: apoptosis and leukocytic infiltration. Intensive Care Med 2010;36:471–478.

23 Duprez L, Takahashi N, Van Hauwermeiren F, Vandendriessche B, Goossens V, Vanden Berghe T, Declercq W, Libert C, Cauwels A, Vandenabeele P: RIP kinase-dependent necrosis drives lethal systemic inflammatory response syndrome. Immunity 2011;35:908–918.

24 Linkermann A, Brasen JH, Himmerkus N, Liu S, Huber TB, Kunzendorf U, Krautwald S: Rip1 (receptor-interacting protein kinase 1) mediates necroptosis and contributes to renal ischemia/reperfusion injury. Kidney Int 2012;81:751–761.

25 Linkermann A, Heller JO, Prokai A, Weinberg JM, De Zen F, Himmerkus N, Szabo AJ, Brasen JH, Kunzendorf U, Krautwald S: The RIP1-kinase inhibitor necrostatin-1 prevents osmotic nephrosis and contrast-induced AKI in mice. J Am Soc Nephrol 2013;24:1545–1557.

26 Brealey D, Brand M, Hargreaves I, Heales S, Land J, Smolenski R, Davies NA, Cooper CE, Singer M: Association between mitochondrial dysfunction and severity and outcome of septic shock. Lancet 2002;360:219–223.

27 Gunst J, Derese I, Aertgeerts A, Ververs EJ, Wauters A, Van den Berghe G, Vanhorebeek I: Insufficient autophagy contributes to mitochondrial dysfunction, organ failure, and adverse outcome in an animal model of critical illness. Crit Care Med 2013;41:182–194.

28 Singh D, Chander V, Chopra K: Cyclosporine protects against ischemia/reperfusion injury in rat kidneys. Toxicology 2005;207:339–347.

29 Sorokin A: Endothelin signaling and actions in the renal mesangium. Contrib Nephrol 2011;172:50–62.

30 Martensson J, Bellomo R: Are all fluids bad for the kidney? Curr Opin Crit Care 2015;21:292–301.

31 Langenberg C, Wan L, Egi M, May CN, Bellomo R: Renal blood flow in experimental septic acute renal failure. Kidney Int 2006;69:1996–2002.

32 Brenner M, Schaer GL, Mallory DL, Suffredini AF, Parrillo JE: Detection of renal blood flow abnormalities in septic and critically ill patients using a newly designed indwelling thermodilution renal vein catheter. Chest 1990;98:170–179.

33 Prowle JR, Molan MP, Hornsey E, Bellomo R: Measurement of renal blood flow by phase-contrast magnetic resonance imaging during septic acute kidney injury: a pilot investigation. Crit Care Med 2012;40:1768–1776.

34 Zafrani L, Payen D, Azoulay E, Ince C: The microcirculation of the septic kidney. Semin Nephrol 2015;35:75–84.

35 Wong BT, Chan MJ, Glassford NJ, Martensson J, Bion V, Chai SY, Oughton C, Tsuji IY, Candal CL, Bellomo R: Mean arterial pressure and mean perfusion pressure deficit in septic acute kidney injury. J Crit Care DOI: 10.1016/j.jcrc.2015.05.003.

36 Asfar P, Meziani F, Hamel JF, Grelon F, Megarbane B, Anguel N, Mira JP, Dequin PF, Gergaud S, Weiss N, et al: High versus low blood-pressure target in patients with septic shock. N Engl J Med 2014;370:1583–1593.

37 Bihari S, Prakash S, Bersten AD: Post resuscitation fluid boluses in severe sepsis or septic shock: prevalence and efficacy (price study). Shock 2013;40:28–34.

38 Glassford NJ, Eastwood GM, Bellomo R: Physiological changes after fluid bolus therapy in sepsis: a systematic review of contemporary data. Crit Care 2014;18:696.

39 Chowdhury AH, Cox EF, Francis ST, Lobo DN: A randomized, controlled, double-blind crossover study on the effects of 2-L infusions of 0.9% saline and plasma-lyte(R) 148 on renal blood flow velocity and renal cortical tissue perfusion in healthy volunteers. Ann Surg 2012;256:18–24.

40 Payen D, de Pont AC, Sakr Y, Spies C, Reinhart K, Vincent JL: A positive fluid balance is associated with a worse outcome in patients with acute renal failure. Crit Care 2008;12:R74.

41 Grams ME, Estrella MM, Coresh J, Brower RG, Liu KD: Fluid balance, diuretic use, and mortality in acute kidney injury. Clin J Am Soc Nephrol 2011;6:966–973.

42 Bouchard J, Soroko SB, Chertow GM, Himmelfarb J, Ikizler TA, Paganini EP, Mehta RL: Fluid accumulation, survival and recovery of kidney function in critically ill patients with acute kidney injury. Kidney Int 2009;76:422–427.

43 Legrand M, Dupuis C, Simon C, Gayat E, Mateo J, Lukaszewicz AC, Payen D: Association between systemic hemodynamics and septic acute kidney injury in critically ill patients: a retrospective observational study. Crit Care 2013;17:R278.

44 Damman K, van Deursen VM, Navis G, Voors AA, van Veldhuisen DJ, Hillege HL: Increased central venous pressure is associated with impaired renal function and mortality in a broad spectrum of patients with cardiovascular disease. J Am Coll Cardiol 2009;53:582–588.

45 Mullens W, Abrahams Z, Francis GS, Sokos G, Taylor DO, Starling RC, Young JB, Tang WH: Importance of venous congestion for worsening of renal function in advanced decompensated heart failure. J Am Coll Cardiol 2009;53:589–596.

Professor Rinaldo Bellomo
Department of Intensive Care
Austin Health
Heidelberg, Vic. 3084 (Australia)
E-Mail rinaldo.bellomo@austin.org.au

# Biomarkers for Diagnosis, Prognosis and Intervention in Acute Kidney Injury

Dana Y. Fuhrman · John A. Kellum

Center for Critical Care Nephrology, Department of Critical Care Medicine, University of Pittsburgh, School of Medicine, Pittsburgh, Pa., USA

## Abstract

Biomarkers for acute kidney injury (AKI) can be used for diagnosis and prognosis and to guide therapy. With no pharmacologic therapy clinically available for the treatment of AKI, prevention and early detection are of paramount importance. Despite the initial enthusiasm for biomarker use when it was first introduced in the literature, published studies' results have shown variability in biomarker performance. The following chapter will discuss what our expectations of AKI biomarkers should be and how they can be currently used for a variety of clinical purposes.

© 2016 S. Karger AG, Basel

## The Use of Biomarkers to Aid in Making a Diagnosis of Acute Kidney Injury

The Kidney Disease Improving Global Outcomes (KDIGO) criteria provide us with specific changes in creatinine and urine output in order to make a diagnosis of acute kidney injury (AKI) [1]. Although serum creatinine remains a useful test for determining that a change in kidney function has occurred, we know that it is a late marker of kidney injury. Given that even small changes in serum creatinine are associated with increased mortality in hospitalized patients, we are in need of markers to detect AKI faster [2]. Effective use of biomarkers requires an understanding of their limitations and individual performance characteristics. Since a certain biomarker may be sensitive to or specific for AKI at a given cutoff, but not both, establishing cutoffs for high sensitivity and high specificity is necessary prior to biomarker use [3].

Additionally, knowledge of the optimal timing for obtaining biomarker values is important. A challenge in the interpretation of biomarker data for predicting AKI occurs in deciding when to evaluate a change in function. Significant changes in function may be missed if biomarkers are checked too early or too late. If a biomarker is obtained prior to a time of functional decline or during a time of functional recovery, the injury could be missed. A common clinical scenario ensues when an individual has an intact renal functional reserve and an injury occurs that is not severe enough to lead to a change in renal function. In this case, the biomarker result will be deemed a 'false positive'. In the interpretation of biomarkers, it is important to understand that an absence of functional change does not rule out injury [3].

Although the specific changes in serum creatinine and urine output provided by the KDIGO criteria give us objective data for defining AKI, making a diagnosis of AKI requires careful clinical judgment before applying the criteria to a patient [4]. There are frequent patient scenarios where the baseline creatinine may not be available or a patient has been given a large volume of fluid, whereby using serum creatinine changes to reflect acute changes in the glomerular filtration rate (GFR) will be difficult or impossible. Certain patient populations have been shown to be more susceptible to AKI, such as those with chronic kidney disease (CKD), diabetes mellitus, malignancies, or an age greater than 65 [5]. Additionally, exposures such as sepsis, critical illness, shock, trauma, cardiac surgery requiring cardiopulmonary bypass, and recent administration of nephrotoxic drugs or radiocontrast agents can all put a patient at increased risk for AKI [6, 7]. When used in the setting of a patient phenotype that may be more at risk for AKI, serum and renal biomarkers can be helpful in making a diagnosis of AKI, especially in cases where the diagnosis is unclear.

Biomarkers along with clinical judgment may useful for determining the likelihood that a patient will develop AKI in the next 24 hours. However, undirected biomarker use with no regard for a specific clinical context is likely to be associated with poor predictive performance for the biomarker. The majority of studies in which biomarkers have a poor capacity to diagnose AKI include more heterogeneous patient populations, as opposed to the stronger biomarker performance cited in studies involving more homogenous patient groups [8]. For example, neutrophil gelatinase-associated lipocalin (NGAL) has been shown to be highly predictive of AKI in pediatric populations undergoing cardiopulmonary bypass [9–12]. Goldstein and Chawla [13] introduced the renal angina concept in 2010 to direct biomarker assessment based on a predetermined risk for AKI. A bedside calculation, termed the 'renal angina index' and including a combination of patient risk factors and signs of injury, predicted severe AKI 3 days after admission in critically ill patients [14]. The authors propose that a risk assessment score such as the renal angina index should be used to allocate the use of biomarkers to patient groups at greater risk for AKI.

## The Use of Biomarkers to Determine Renal Prognosis in Acute Kidney Injury

The ability of biomarkers to predict CKD progression or renal recovery has been investigated. For example, when NGAL was evaluated in patients with community-acquired pneumonia on the first day that they experienced severe AKI, NGAL was useful for predicting renal recovery, defined as being alive, not requiring dialysis during hospitalization or having a persistent RIFLE-F classification at the time of hospital discharge [15].

The concept of acute kidney disease, defined as a GFR less than 60 ml/min per 1.73 m$^2$ or evidence of structural kidney damage for less than 3 months, was proposed by the KDIGO AKI Workgroup [1]. These patients may present with a seemingly normal serum creatinine and an absence of proteinuria but are at a high risk for multiple AKI events and rapid progression to CKD given certain susceptibilities and exposures. Biomarkers may play a role in predicting the AKI-to-CKD transition. Partial recovery after an episode of AKI very likely has a worse prognosis when compared to complete recovery. We know that AKI with apparent complete recovery confers an increased risk for CKD development [16]. Biomarkers may be useful for predicting renal recovery (or a lack thereof) in those individuals who, based on our currently available clinical assessment tools, seem to have achieved renal recovery.

Newer biomarkers, including urinary tissue inhibitor of metalloproteinase-2 (TIMP-2) and insulin-like growth factor-binding protein 7 (IGFBP7), may fill this role. TIMP-2 and IGFBP7 are markers of G1 cell cycle arrest that are expressed in tubular cells in response to DNA damage [17, 18]. By initiating cell cycle arrest, cells can avoid division during times of stress or injury, which is protective [19]. In contrast to many previously studied biomarkers, which act as a signal for cellular injury, TIMP-2 and IGFBP7 increase in response to a wide variety of insults and potentially act as signals for early cellular stress [19]. These markers have been validated for risk assessment for AKI in critically ill patients [20, 21]. Interestingly, in a secondary analysis of a prospective observational study of critically ill adults, Koyner et al. [22] found that in those with AKI, a [TIMP-2]·[IGFBP7] value (the product of TIMP-2 and IGFBP7 levels) greater than 2 (ng/ml)$^2$/1,000 was associated with increased mortality or a need for renal replacement therapy over the next 9 months (hazard ratio, 2.16; 95% CI, 1.32–3.53; $p = 0.002$).

Unlike in other organ systems, kidney dysfunction may evolve silently until overt renal failure occurs. We know that in a healthy human, more than 50% of renal function must be lost before serum creatinine rises. Having a method to predict which patients are more likely to develop rapidly progressive renal disease and show a greater-than-age-dependent decline in the GFR would prove invaluable when faced with patients who are at a high risk for numerous renal insults during a hospital or lifetime course. In practice, clinicians will frequently attribute a rapid rise in serum creatinine that is out of proportion to what would be expected following a seemingly small renal insult to a loss of or decrease in renal reserve filtration capacity. Bosch et al. [23] first introduced the concept of renal reserve for clinical use in the 1980s, when they did a group of studies examining the effects of protein loading on the GFR. They defined renal reserve as the difference between the stimulated GFR and the baseline GFR. Healthy individuals have an average increase of 32 ml/min × 1.73 m$^2$ (10–30%) in their GFR 1–3 hours after a protein load [23–26]. However, we currently do not have an easy way to clinically measure renal reserve. Previous methods have relied on renal clearance methods that require timed urine collections, which can be technically challenging and inaccurate [27]. Cystatin C, a protease inhibitor and rapidly responsive biomarker, was found to increase significantly after a meat meal in healthy young adults [28]. Given that cystatin C has a relatively short half-life, with levels that respond rapidly to changes in the GFR, its assessment may be a convenient method for measuring renal reserve in those thought to be at risk for progression to CKD.

Similar to the way that we measure the response of the heart and lungs to increased physiologic demand with cardiac and pulmonary exercise testing, might renal biomarkers aid us in quantifying renal fitness? A kidney with a lack of fitness may be operating at its maximal filtration capacity and have no ability to increase its GFR in response to a stimulus or stressor. There are many patient populations, such as oncology and cardiac patients, that are exposed to numerous predictable and often preventable renal insults during the course of treatment. Biomarkers could potentially provide an early risk stratification of renal fitness for these patients. Chronically elevated levels of TIMP-2 and IGFBP7 may indicate ongoing cellular stress and a lack of renal fitness. Furthermore, might an inability to increase the levels of markers of cellular stress during times of renal insult indicate a maladaptive response?

For example, consider two 26-year-old female patients with congenital heart disease and a history of staged operative repair (fig. 1). At baseline, Patient 1 has a renal functional reserve of 25%, whereas Patient 2 has a renal function reserve of 6%. At an outpatient clinic visit, both patients have a serum creatinine of 0.8 mg/dl, normal blood pressure and no proteinuria. They have both been

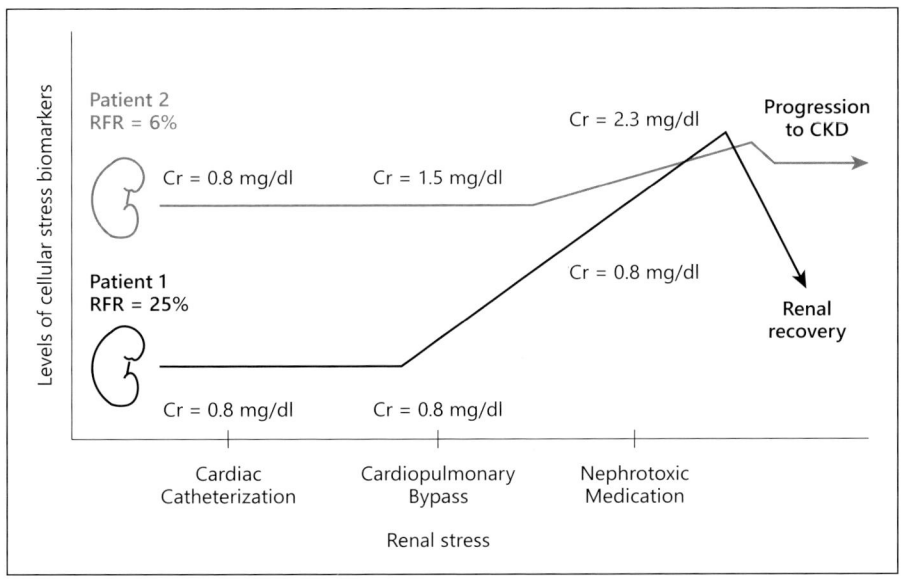

**Fig. 1.** Baseline renal reserve and levels of cellular stress biomarkers may predict the response to renal stress.

experiencing symptoms of heart failure and are therefore admitted for cardiac catheterization. Both patients subsequently need operative intervention requiring cardiopulmonary bypass, and both patients receive nephrotoxic medications peri-operatively. Even though both patients exhibit injury to their kidneys, creatinine levels remain unchanged for Patient 1, whereas there is a significant increase following the cardiac catheterization in Patient 2. Their courses also differ in that Patient 2 progresses to CKD and Patient 1 experiences full renal recovery. As in the case of Patient 2, a kidney that is in a consistent state of maximal filtration capacity and cellular stress will likely be unable to respond to external stressors by increasing the GFR. Note that subclinical 'stress' on the organ, depicted on the y-axis, is also different. While Patient 1 experiences significant stress, she has sufficient reserve to avoid experiencing decreased function. Conversely, Patient 2 is already in a state of high stress/low reserve, and the exposures result in a marked change in function. Might these patients also differ in terms of cellular injury? At present, it is unknown, but it is intriguing to speculate that renal fitness might entail not only the ability to call on reserve function when some nephrons become injured but also possibly resistance to injury in the first place. Various cellular adaptions, from down-regulation in energy use to cell cycle arrest, could provide the mechanistic links for this concept. If these patients could be identified early, before injury, interventions to support renal recovery could be implemented, such as avoidance of nephrotoxic medications, careful attention to fluid management, and close follow-up by a nephrologist after hospital discharge to potentially avoid progression to CKD, or failing this, to at least treat the CKD as early as possible. We speculate that [TIMP-2]·[IGFBP7] might serve as a useful marker of renal stress and may ultimately be used for this purpose. However, much additional work is needed before this approach can be used clinically.

**Biomarkers and Therapeutic Intervention for Acute Kidney Injury**

Although we do not have direct therapeutic agents available for the treatment of AKI at the present time, there are ongoing studies exploring potential future therapies. Biomarkers may be useful in selecting patients who might better respond to treatment modalities for AKI. For example, the AKI incidence was significantly reduced in 240 adult patients at very high risk for AKI who underwent cardiac surgery and were randomized to receive remote ischemic preconditioning (RIPC) with upper-arm blood pressure cuff inflations prior to surgery when compared to a control group [29]. When measured prior to cardiopulmonary bypass, [TIMP-2]·[IGFBP7] increased in the majority of patients receiving RIPC. Additionally, in those who had an increase in [TIMP-2]·[IGFBP7] after RIPC and prior to cardiopulmonary bypass, the incidence of AKI was reduced compared to the incidence in those who did not [29]. This suggests that increases in biomarkers may be used to predict which patients will respond to RIPC, a potential therapeutic intervention for the prevention of AKI. The important differences that exist between biomarker-positive versus biomarker-negative individuals may likely dictate a predicted response to therapy.

In the case of clinical trials, biomarkers could be used to exclude those participants at low risk for an outcome, to enrich the study population sampled, and therefore to increase the event rate. Selecting out low-risk subjects could lead to a lower required sample size to detect a significant study difference [3]. Using biomarkers to aid in the selection of a higher-risk patient group for a study could lead to a focus on those more likely to benefit from an intervention. Similarly, the use of enrichment is also important clinically since efforts to improve clinical outcomes will be most effective when focused on the highest-risk groups [30].

**Conclusion**

The addition of AKI biomarkers to clinical judgment along with knowledge of clinically meaningful cutoffs and the optimal timing of acquisition has great potential for improving biomarkers' diagnostic capabilities. It is likely that in the future, biomarkers will be useful not only for predicting an impending AKI event but also for anticipating a kidney's response to an 'AKI exposure' and an individual's renal prognosis after AKI. Biomarkers will likely have an important role in clinical trial design as we move toward discovering and developing therapeutic interventions for a complex syndrome like AKI.

## References

1 KDIGO AKI Workgroup. Kidney disease: improving global outcomes (KDIGO) clinical practice guideline for acute kidney injury. Kidney Int Suppl 2012;2:1–141.
2 Chertow GM, Burdick E, Honour M, et al: Acute kidney injury, mortality, length of stay, and costs in hospitalized patients. J Am Soc Nephol 2005;16:3365–3370.
3 Kellum JA, Devarajan P: What can we expect from biomarkers for acute kidney injury? Biomark Med 2014;8:1239–1245.
4 Kellum JA, Bellomo R, Ronco C: Does this patient have acute kidney injury? An AKI checklist. Intensive Care Med DOI: 10.1007/s00134-015-4026-4.
5 Hoste EAJ, Bagshaw SM, Bellamo R, et al: Epidemiology of acute kidney injury in critically ill patients: the multinational AKI-EPI study. Intensive Care Med 2015;8:1411–1423.
6 Sileanu FE, Murugan R, Lucko N, et al: AKI in low-risk versus high-risk patients in the intensive care. Clin J Am Soc Nephrol 2014;6:187–196.
7 Qianyi P, Lina Z, Yuhang A, et al: Epidemiology of acute kidney injury in intensive care septic patients based on the KDIGO guidelines. Chin Med J 2014;127:1820–1826.
8 Chawla LS, Goldstein SL, Kellum JA, Ronco C: Renal angina: concept and development of pretest probability assessment in acute kidney injury. Crit Care 2015;19:93–97.
9 Mishra J, Dent C, Tarabishi R, et al: Neutrophil gelatinase-associated lipocalin (NGAL) as a biomarker for acute renal injury after cardiac surgery. Lancet 2005;365:1231–1238.
10 Bennett M, Dent CL, Ma Q, et al: Urine NGAL predicts severity of acute kidney injury after cardiac surgery: a prospective study. Clin J Am Soc Nephrol 2008;3:665–673.
11 Dent CI, Ma Q, Dastrala S, et al: Plasma neutrophil gelatinase-associated lipocalin predicts acute kidney injury, morbidity and mortality after pediatric cardiac surgery: a prospective uncontrolled cohort study. Crit Care 2007;11:R27.
12 Krawczeski CD, Woo JG, Wang Y, et al: Neutrophil gelatinase-associated lipocalin concentrations predict development of acute kidney injury in neonates and children after cardiopulmonary bypass. J Pediatr 2011;158:1009–1015.
13 Goldstein SL, Chawla LS: Renal angina. Clin J Am Soc Nephrol 2011;5:943–949.
14 Basu RK, Zappitelli M, Brunner L, et al: Derivation and validation of the renal angina index to improve the prediction of acute kidney injury in critically ill children. Kidney Int 2013;85:659–667.
15 Srsawat N, Murugan R, Lee M, et al: Genetic inflammatory markers of sepsis study I: plasma neutrophil gelatinase-associated lipocalin predicts recovery from acute kidney injury following community-acquired pneumonia. Kidney Int 2001;80:545–552.
16 Hsu CY, Ordonez JD, Chertow GM, et al: The risk of acute renal failure in patients with chronic kidney disease. Kidney Int 2008;74:101–107.
17 Seo DW, Li H, Qu CK, et al: Shp-1 mediates the antiproliferative activity of tissue inhibitor of metalloproteinase-2 in human microvascular endothelial cells. J Biol Chem 2006;281:3711–3721.
18 Zuo S, Liu C, Wang J: IGFBP-rP1 induces p21 expression through a p53-independent pathway, leading to cellular senscence of MCF-7 breast cancer cells. J Cancer Res Clin Oncol 2012;138:1045–1055.
19 Devarajan P: Update on mechanisms of ischemic acute kidney injury. J Am Soc Nephron 2006;17:1503–1520.

20 Kashani K, Al-Khafaji A, Ardiles T, et al: Discovery and validation of cell cycle arrest biomarkers in human acute kidney injury. Crit Care 2013;17:R25.
21 Bihorac A, Chawla LS, Shaw AD, et al: Validation of cell-cycle arrest biomarkers for acute kidney injury using clinical adjudication. Am J Respir Crit Care Med 2014;189: 932–939.
22 Koyner JL, Shaw AD, Chawla LS: Tissue inhibitor metalloproteinase-2 (TIMP-2) IGF-Binding Protein-7 (IGFBP7) levels are associated with adverse long-term outcomes in patients with AKI. JASN 2015;26:1747–1754.
23 Bosch JP, Saccaggi A, Lauer A, et al: Renal functional reserve in humans. Effect of protein intake on glomerular filtration rate. Am J Med 1983;75:943–950.
24 Solling K, Christensen CK, Solling J, et al: Effect on renal haemodynamics, glomerular filtration rate and albumin excretion of high oral protein load. Scand J Clin Lab Invest 1986;46:351–357.
25 Rodriguez-Iturbe B, Herrera J, Garcia R: Relationship between glomerular filtration rate and renal blood flow at different levels of protein induced filtration in man. Clin Sci 1988;74:11–15.
26 Hostetter TH: Human renal response to a meat meal. Am J Physiol 1986;250:F613–F618.
27 Schwartz GJ, Work DF: Measurement and estimation of GFR in children and adolescents. Clin J Am Soc Nephrol 2009;4:1832–1843.
28 Fuhrman DY, Maier PS, Schwartz GJ: Rapid assessment of renal reserve in young adults by cystatin C. Scand J Clin Lab Invest 2013; 73:265–268.
29 Zarbock A, Schmidt C, Van Aken H, et al: Effect of remote ischemic preconditioning on kidney injury among high-risk patients undergoing cardiac surgery. JAMA 2015;313: 2133–2141.
30 Kellum JA, Chawla LS: Cell-cycle arrest and acute kidney injury: the light and the dark sides. Nephrol Dial Transplant DOI: 10.1093/ndt/gfv130.

John A. Kellum, MD, MCCM
Center for Critical Care Nephrology, Department of Critical Care Medicine
University of Pittsburgh, 604 Scaife Hall, 3550 Terrace Street
Pittsburgh, PA 15261 (USA)
E-Mail kellumja@ccm.upmc.edu

# The Acute Kidney Injury to Chronic Kidney Disease Transition: A Potential Opportunity to Improve Care in Acute Kidney Injury

Carlos E. Palant[a, c] · Richard L. Amdur[b, e] · Lakhmir S. Chawla[a, c, d]

[a]Department of Medicine, and [b]Biostatistics Core Laboratory, Veterans Affairs Medical Center, [c]Division of Renal Diseases and Hypertension, Department of Medicine and Departments of [d]Anesthesiology and Critical Care Medicine and [e]Surgery, George Washington University Medical Center, Washington, D.C., USA

## Abstract

Recent controlled trials, epidemiological analyses and basic research studies offer a comprehensive view of the short and long-term clinical repercussion of de novo acute kidney injury or AKI. While most post-AKI patients recover their baseline renal function, a significant number, approximately ~20% of those affected, will go on to develop long term illness characterized by an increase in late stage CKD, cardiovascular complications, and increased death rates. When AKI occurs in hospitalized patients, selected demographic and laboratory results can be incorporated into risk calculators that identify those at higher risk for long-term complications. This review touches on some of the salient epidemiological studies of the AKI to CKD transition. It also focuses on certain recent advancements in our understanding of the biological and functional impact of AKI on the renal tubule repair mechanism, as well as the important role that genetic, epigenetic, biochemical and inflammatory events, seemingly beneficial to the re-establishment of normal renal function, can be offset by mediators of progressive fibrosis and irreversible structural changes. Characterization of basic processes that mediate the AKI to CKD transition reveals promising pharmacological and biological agents that hopefully will one day be used in the early stages of AKI to prevent its deadly consequences.

© 2016 S. Karger AG, Basel

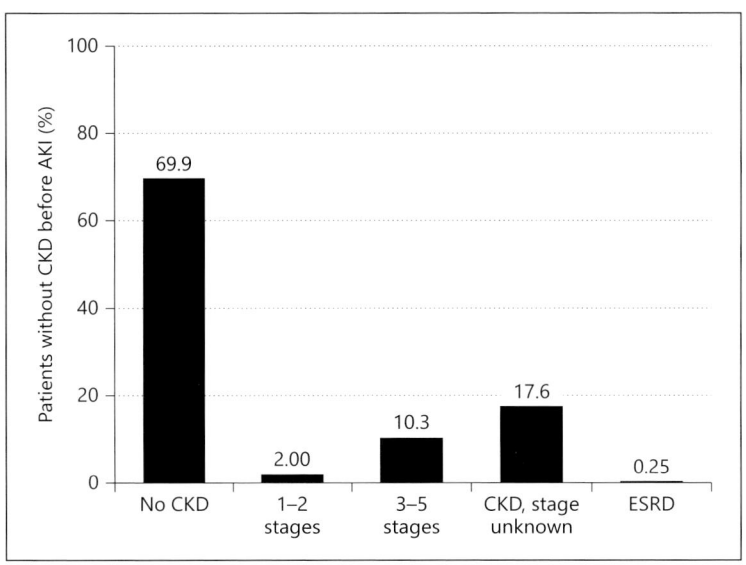

**Fig. 1.** Renal statuses at 1 year following discharge from AKI hospitalization from 2010 to 2011 of surviving Medicare patients aged 66+ without kidney disease prior to AKI hospitalization, grouped by CKD stage and ESRD status. Data source: Medicare 5% sample. The Medicare patients were aged 66 and older and had both Medicare Parts A & B, no Medicare Advantage plan (Part C/HMO), did not have ESRD, were discharged alive from a first AKI hospitalization in 2010 or 2011, and did not have any claims with a diagnosis of CKD in the 365 days prior to AKI. Renal status after AKI was determined from claims reported between discharge from AKI hospitalization and 365 days after discharge. Stage was determined by the 585.x claim reported the closest to 365 days after discharge, and ESRD was determined by the first service date listed on the Medical Evidence form. AKI = Acute kidney injury; CKD = chronic kidney disease; ESRD = end-stage renal disease. Reprinted with permission from [2].

## Epidemiology of the Acute Kidney Injury-Chronic Kidney Disease Interconnection

The incidence of acute kidney injury (AKI) is estimated at 2,147 cases per million population per year [1]. Given the US population of 300 million, each year, there will be ~600,000 cases of AKI. If 20% of such patients progress to advanced chronic kidney disease (CKD), then there will be 120,000 annual cases of CKD caused by AKI. Figure 1 depicts a Medicare cohort [2] at 1 year following discharge from AKI hospitalization from 2010 to 2011, including surviving patients aged 66 and older without kidney disease prior to AKI hospitalization, grouped by CKD and end-stage renal disease (ESRD) status. Among these AKI patients aged 66 and older, in 2012, fewer than 50% were discharged to their home. The mortality rate (including discharge to hospice) was 14.4%, while 29.7% of the patients were discharged to institutions, including short-term skilled nursing facilities, rehabilitation hospitals and long-term care facilities (USRDS 2014). In addition, AKI is an independent risk factor for cardiovascular morbidity [3] and a shortened life span [4]. Therefore, careful examination of the AKI-CKD relationship has highly significant clinical and public health implications. For over 50 years, AKI was considered by clinician-scholars as a reversible syndrome, although early publications, which were limited by the sizes of the populations examined, indicated that a significant number of post-AKI patients suffered permanent loss of renal function [5–16]. Lack of longitudinal measurements of renal function, failure to exclude patients with pre-existing renal disease, and use of small populations (i.e. studies from single centers) limited full assessments of renal and patient survival during the post-AKI period. Given that aging may be associated with a decline in the glomerular filtration rate, it is critical to compare renal survival in post-AKI patients with demographically similar patients with no evidence of a past episode of AKI. More recently, the availability of large institutional databases has enabled investigators to retrospectively examine clinical trajectories of post-AKI patients with respect to risk factors for progression to CKD, mortality rates compared to age-matched controls, and the independent effects of AKI on nonrenal outcomes. Consensus definitions for grading the severity of AKI (RIFLE, AKIN, and KDIGO) identify AKI survivors that are most likely to progress to advanced CKD stages, although studies have demonstrated that that even mild [17] and reversible AKI [18] are associated with adverse short- and long-term outcomes. Last but not least, it is also critical to rank AKI among other life-threatening illnesses with a high cardiovascular disease or inflammatory burden so that its impact on the health of the public at large can be adequately assessed.

Over the last 20 years or so, electronic health records have allowed for numerous retrospective epidemiological studies to be performed examining both short- and long-term outcomes of AKI in terms of progression to CKD and mortality (see below), as well as other outcomes [3, 4]. Using a large Veterans Affairs database of patients hospitalized between 1999 and 2005, our group compared rates of renal and patient survival for patients hospitalized with *de novo* AKI (i.e. no history of previous AKI and normal baseline estimated glomerular filtration rate (GFR) with those for patients who suffered from acute myocardial infarction (MI) or an episode of pneumonia (PNE) [19]. Figures 2–4 summarize some of our findings as Kaplan-Meier plots of renal and patient survival estimates of time in months from in-patient ICD-9 diagnosis of acute tubular necrosis (ATN) and acute renal failure (ARF), with comparisons of two groups, CKD patients (mean estimated GFR of <60 ml/min/1.73 m$^2$

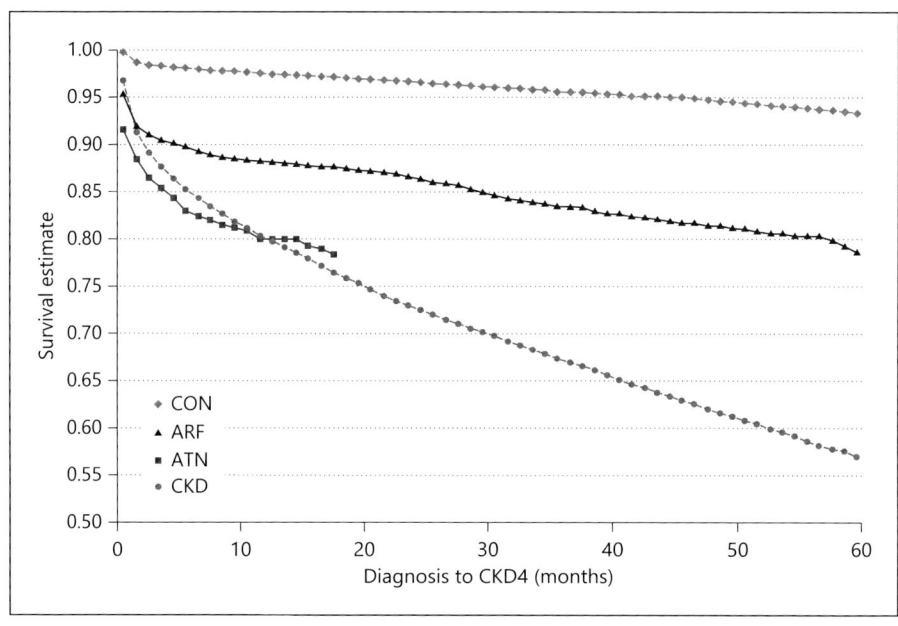

**Fig. 2.** Kaplan-Meier survival estimates of time (months) from diagnosis to entry into CKD stage 4 according to subject type. CKD subjects who had already developed CKD4 prior to their diagnosis date are not included.

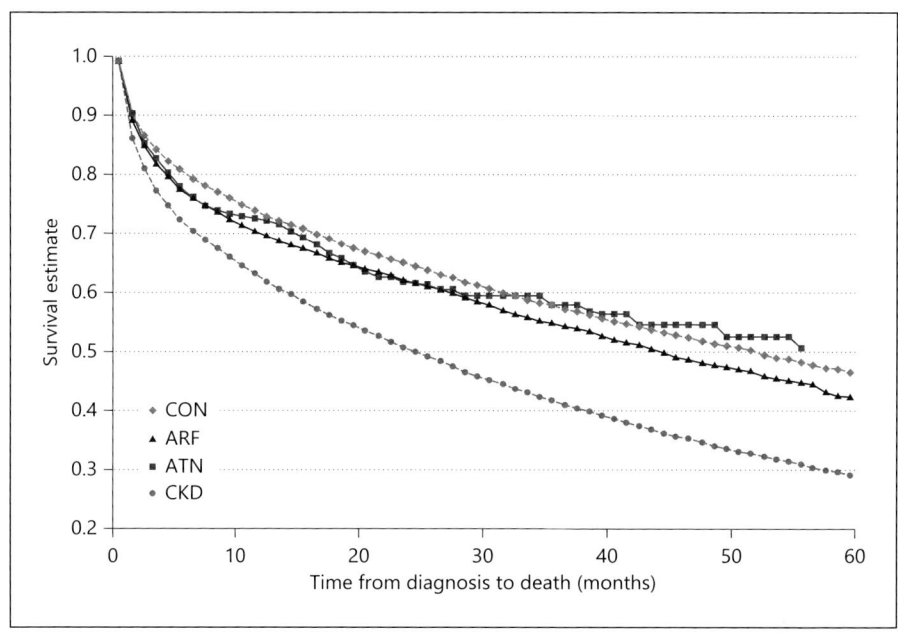

**Fig. 3.** Kaplan-Meier survival estimates of time (months) from diagnosis to death according to subject type.

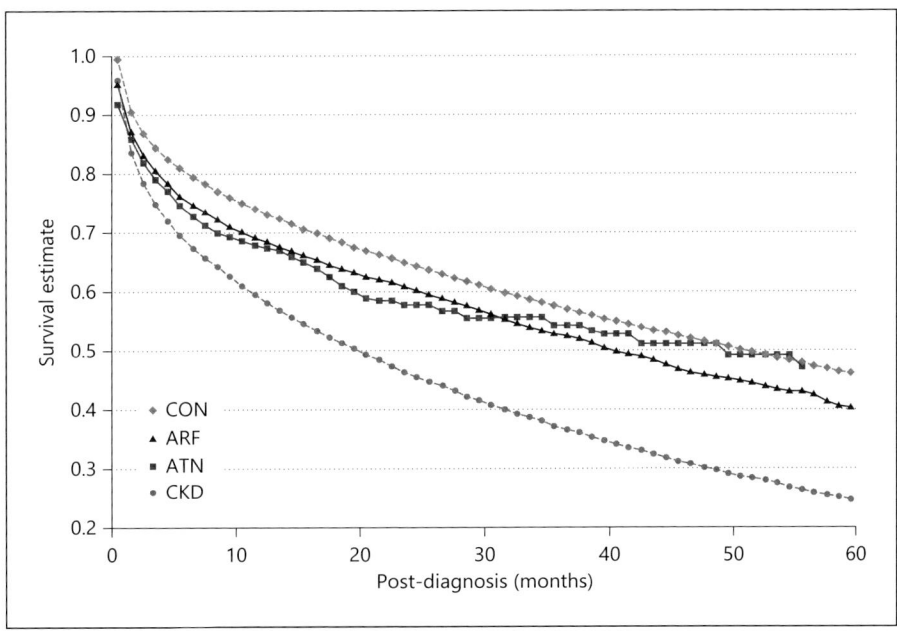

**Fig. 4.** Kaplan-Meier survival estimates of time (months) from diagnosis to combined endpoint (the earliest of CKD4, chronic dialysis, or death) according to subject type.

during the year before their admission date) and patients hospitalized for either an episode of PNE or MI (controls or CON) without known prior kidney disease. Figure 2 illustrates survival from diagnosis to entry into stage 4 CKD, figure 3 illustrates survival in months from diagnosis to death, and figure 4 shows the time from diagnosis to a combined endpoint of CKD4, chronic dialysis or death. The sample size for this study was as follows: 5,021 patients with ARF, 345 with ATN, 62,650 patients in the CON group, and 44,076 patients in the CKD group. Of note, all diagnoses of ATN and ARF as well as CKD were validated by serum creatinine (SC) measurements and corrected for multiple co-morbidities. This study has confirmed that AKI constitutes a significant factor for progression to CKD in about 20% of patients with *de novo* AKI. Several contemporaneous studies with generally similar objectives as ours were recently summarized by Coca et al. [20] in a systematic review and meta-analysis of studies examining AKI to CKD progression. Using electronic databases, web search engines, and bibliographies, 13 cohort studies were selected (table 1). For individuals who had suffered from an episode of AKI, the pooled incidence rates of CKD and ESRD were 25.8 per 100 person-years and 8.6 per 100 person-years, respectively. The AKI patients had a pooled adjusted hazard ratio (HR) for the development of CKD of 8.8, (95% CI 3.1–

**Table 1.** Meta-analysis of CKD and ESRD associated with AKI. Adapted from Coca et al. [20]

| Study or subgroup | Weight (%) | HR IV, random, 95% CI |
|---|---|---|
| (a) Pooled adjusted HRs for CKD after AKI | | |
| Weiss et al. [70] | 10.0 | 32.79 (4.30–249.77) |
| Amdur et al. [19] | 15.5 | 6.64 (5.05–8.74) |
| Lo et al. [21] | 15.5 | 28.08 (21.01–37.53) |
| James et al. [22] | 15.6 | 29.99 (24.32–36.99) |
| James et al. [10, 11] | 15.5 | 1.60 (1.20–2.14) |
| Ando et al. [71] | 12.4 | 9.91 (2.48–39.63) |
| Ishani et al. [23] | 15.6 | 2.33 (1.83–2.96) |
| Total [95% CI] | 100.0 | 8.82 (3.05–25.48) |
| (b) Pooled adjusted HRs for ESRD after AKI | | |
| Newsome et al. [12] | 15.0 | 3.26 (2.87–3.70) |
| Ishani et al. [23] | 14.8 | 12.99 (10.57–15.96) |
| Wald et al. [13] | 14.9 | 3.22 (2.70–3.85) |
| Hsu et al. [23] | 13.5 | 1.47 (0.95–2.28) |
| James et al. [10, 11] | 12.5 | 4.15 (2.32–7.41) |
| Lafrance et al. [15] | 15.0 | 2.33 (2.08–2.61) |
| Choi et al. [16] | 14.4 | 1.37 (1.02–1.84) |
| Total (95% CI) | 100.0 | 3.10 (1.91–5.03) |

25.5), a pooled adjusted HR for ESRD of 3.1 (95% CI 1.9–5.0), and a pooled adjusted mortality HR of 2.0 (95% CI 1.3–3.1) compared to the patients without AKI. Of particular interest, two of the studies that examined AKI outcomes in patients with pre-existing CKD found that the relative risk for the development of CKD and ESRD was higher than that in patients without pre-existing CKD [21, 22]. This result was somewhat unexpected given that patients with compromised renal function should be the least able to tolerate an acute renal insult. In fact, using a Medicare database, Ishani et al. [23] demonstrated that pre-existing CKD was a significant risk factor for developing ESRD among patients hospitalized with AKI. However, this study relied exclusively on the End-Stage Renal Disease Medical Evidence Report (CMS-2728), a cross-sectional examination of Medicare data, and did not provide information on level of CKD severity. Several other studies have also emphasized the role of CKD as a risk factor for AKI (table 2). More recently, two large meta-analyses have offered compelling evidence that CKD is a major risk factor for AKI, surpassing the effects of age, diabetes mellitus, and hypertension (HTN) but not those of albuminuria [24, 25]. Elucidation of the link between AKI and CKD will require additional prospective trials of post-AKI patients. Initial evidence obtained by closely monitoring dialysis-requiring AKI patients in a short-term

**Table 2.** Causes of AKI: exposures and susceptibilities for non-specific AKI

| Exposures | Susceptibilities |
|---|---|
| Sepsis | Dehydration or volume depletion |
| Critical illness | Advanced age |
| Circulatory shock | Female gender |
| Burns | Black race |
| Trauma | CKD |
| Cardiac surgery (especially with CPB) | Chronic diseases (heart, lung, liver) |
| Major noncardiac surgery | Diabetes mellitus |
| Nephrotoxic drugs | Cancer |
| Radiocontrast agents | Anemia |
| Poisonous plants and animals | |

CPB = Cardiopulmonary bypass. Adapted from KDIGO 2015 [27].

prospective follow-up trial is not encouraging because it shows that recovery of renal function occurs in less than 25% of patients at 28 days of follow-up [26].

Multiple risk factors for AKI have been established. A recent review of factors that predispose patient to AKI, conducted by KDIGO scholars based on several published manuscripts, is presented in table 2 [27]. In our recent study on the outcomes of AKI, bedside equations were formulated that may be able to predict the probability of progression to late-stage CKD in post-AKI patients with a high degree of accuracy [28], although these equations require validation by other investigators in different patient populations.

Our previous study [28] examined predictors of entry into stage 4 CKD over a mean of 2.4 ± 1.6 years in a model development sample of 5,351 US veterans without pre-existing CKD who were admitted with a primary AKI diagnosis over a 5-year period. We then used the prediction model developed for that sample in a separate validation sample of 15,917 control patients who also had no pre-existing CKD and were admitted during the same time frame, with a primary diagnosis of either MI or PNE and data on the R, I, or F RIFLE scores (i.e. the patients in the validation group also had AKI, as indicated by their SC levels at admission). A primary risk prediction model, as well as two simplified models using variables that are readily available to clinicians, were developed and were then independently validated. For all three models, the c-statistics showed good discrimination in the derivation sample (c = ~0.80), with little or no reduction in the validation sample. For a range of risk score cut points, sensitivity and specificity showed small decreases in the validation sample relative to the development sample, indicating that these models would likely work well for use in similar patient populations. Further validation would be helpful, especially for female patients with AKI.

The primary prediction model included age, diabetes mellitus, mean SC level at admission, African-American race, mean serum albumin (SA) level over a 1-year baseline period prior to hospitalization, and mean SA level at admission. However, a simpler model worked nearly as well using just age, mean SC level at admission, and mean SA level at admission (c = 0.81 in both the test and validation samples). The risk equation that would be used clinically based on this model is as follows: Risk = 0.0162 x age + 0.3655 x (mean SC during admission) – 1.1468 x (mean SA during admission). If a single risk cut point is used, then in the validation sample, a risk score of <–2.25 indicates a lower risk of CKD4, while a risk score of ≥–2.25 indicates a higher risk.

Similar methods have recently been used in other studies to develop and test prediction models for CKD progression [29–33]. However, these studies have not focused on the AKI patient population, and in general, they have not used separate validation samples.

## Pathophysiology of the Acute Kidney Injury to Chronic Kidney Disease Transition

In recent years, a number of publications [34–45] have reviewed the pathobiology of the AKI and early post-AKI periods. Using mostly rodents as models, ischemia-reperfusion injury (IRI), unilateral ureteral obstruction, and 5/6th nephrectomy have served as paradigms of the early mechanism and pathology of AKI and how the early events may eventually cause the advanced interstitial fibrosis that is characteristic of progression to CKD. Furthermore, these models provide opportunities to explore potentially promising pharmacological and biological approaches aimed at not only repairing necrotic tubular epithelia but also arresting progression to a chronic stage. From these studies, we have learned that following induction of AKI, tubular epithelial cells, vascular endothelial cells, interstitial cells, and blood- and bone marrow-borne cells all participate in a complex and orchestrated but sometimes imperfect process aimed at limiting and subsequently repairing damaged cells and restoring their function. For tubular epithelial cells, this means restoration of cell polarity and tight junctional integrity, which will allow for the return of vectorial electrolyte and nutrient transport and paracrine functions. For vascular endothelial cells, this means restoring adequate blood flow to nephrons, which limits the effects of oxygen and nutrient deprivation and ensures that vascular auto-regulatory mechanisms are reestablished.

Genetic and epigenetic phenomena, humoral mediators of inflammation, such as cytokines, chemokines, microRNAs (miRNAs), damage-associated molecular pattern molecules, growth factors, vasoactive peptides and regulators of cell death, initiate a reparative process that at times runs in tandem or is followed by a noxious sequence in which pro-inflammatory mediators may cause progressive losses of renal mass and function.

*Genetic, Epigenetic and microRNAs Roles in the Acute Kidney Injury to Chronic Kidney Disease Transition*

Within 4 h following experimental AKI, immediate-early genes responsible for tissue repair are up-regulated, including *Fos* (an inducer of cell proliferation, differentiation and survival), *Jun* (a regulator of apoptosis), and *Egr1* (a regulator of cell growth). Within 4–24 h, numerous other molecular indicators are expressed, including hemoxygenase-1 *(Ho-1)*, *Lcn2* (NGAL), *Havcr1* (Kim1), annexin A2 *(Anxa2)*, clusterin, and interleukin 6 *(IL-6)*. HO-1 is of special interest because it acts as a rescue factor that mitigates the oxidative stress resulting from IRI (see below). Several apoptotic genes are up-regulated during this early post-AKI period, including *Fadd, Daxx Bad,* and *Bak,* as well as the anti-apoptotic gene *Bcl2,* which is known to attenuate the adverse effects of IRI. In addition, several genes known to be involved in the tubular repair/regeneration process are expressed, including *Nmyc1* and *Wt1*, as well as *Gdnf* and *Mdk,* which encode growth factors [34].

Basile et al. [46] examined renal tissue from rats 35 days after recovery from bilateral IRI, comparing the gene expression with that in renal tissue obtained from sham-operated rats using a cDNA microarray containing ~2,000 known rat genes. Sixteen genes were identified as persistently altered. The expression of genes associated with fibrosis and calcification, including those encoding osteopontin and matrix Gla protein, was enhanced. The expression of pro-inflammatory genes, including those encoding S100A4, a specific marker for fibroblasts, and complement C4, were also enhanced in post-ischemic tissues. Conversely, kallikrein expression was reduced during the post-ischemic phase.

Activation of genes encoding complement cascade components were also identified by several days following AKI, suggesting the persistence of an inflammatory state, as well as continuous extracellular matrix remodeling [47]. Expression of chemokines (Ccl2, Ccl6, Ccl12, and Ccl17) and monocyte chemoattractant protein 1 has been shown to attract monocytes-macrophages, dendritic cells, memory T cells, and basophils [34, 48]. Although the repair process may be enhanced by these cells during the early stages of post-AKI injury and repair, its persistence may forecast impaired tubular regeneration and eventual tubulo-interstitial fibrosis. Monocytes potentiate injury after ischemia and promote fibroblast proliferation and fibrosis [37], and macrophage depletion reduces TNF-α release locally, attenuating its cytotoxic effects on renal epithelial cells. C57BL/6 mice infused with clodronate to deplete them of macrophages have been shown to be partially protected from AKI following IRI [49].

Epigenetics plays a role in restoration of tubular cell integrity following experimental AKI. This process has been described as the modulation of gene expression via the posttranslational modification of protein complexes associated with DNA without a change in DNA sequence, as well as expression of miRNAs. Acetylation and de-acetylation of histones can either relax or condense chromatin, resulting in either the activation or inhibition of gene expression [50, 51]. Histone acetyltransferase activity is required for epithelial cell proliferation, and up- or down-regulation of DNA acetylation may either stimulate or inhibit cell proliferation [52]. Epigenetic modulation underlies endotoxin-mediated hyper-responsiveness of cytokine production after AKI [53]. Thus, regulation of gene expression through epigenetic events seems to play a crucial role in epithelial regeneration as well as inflammation.

miRNAs are small, highly conserved, noncoding RNA molecules encoded in the genome that regulate the expression of genes by binding to the 3′-untranslated regions of specific mRNAs and acting as post-transcriptional regulators of target mRNA. For example, the silencing of miRNA-24 following IRI has been shown to ameliorate apoptosis and functional abnormalities under hypoxic conditions in renal endothelial and epithelial cells [54]. A mouse model in which proximal tubular cells lack DICER, an enzyme required for miRNA production, are somewhat resistant to IRI [55]. In an animal model of CKD, miRNA-146a expression has been reported to be correlated with tubulo-interstitial inflammation [56]. In a particularly promising experimental therapeutic approach, intravenous injection of miRNAs that modulate cellular proliferation, angiogenesis and apoptosis has been demonstrated to confer renoprotective effects in an IRI model [57]. Thus, further research is needed to examine the adequate balance between various miRNAs that enhance AKI-induced tubular damage in kidneys and those that protect kidneys from this damage. Modulation of miRNA activity should remain an active area of investigation to reveal new therapeutic pathways for the treatment of AKI and its long-term consequences.

*Cellular and Microvascular Events Contribute to the Acute Kidney Injury to Chronic Kidney Disease Transition*
In septic-mediated AKI, the most common form of injury to the proximal renal tubules, epithelial damage-associated molecular pattern molecules are re-

leased during cell necrosis and by the extracellular matrix and are recognized by constitutive Toll-like receptors. This interaction initiates a systemic inflammatory response with both humoral (cytokines and chemokines) and cellular (dendritic cells, macrophages, natural killer cells, and neutrophils) components that has the potential to cause irreparable damage [40]. Experimental work performed by Venkatachalam et al. [37] has delineated critical events following AKI that block the normal regeneration of renal tubular epithelia. These events include the following: failed differentiation of regenerated epithelia, followed by autophagy/apoptosis and eventual tubular atresia; failure of vascular autoregulation and barotrauma to glomerular capillaries following loss of renal mass; capillary rarefaction, which causes additional hypoxic damage to renal tissue; and initiation of interstitial fibrosis. With respect to the latter, a salient finding of the work by these authors is that traditional reversible AKI is usually associated with self-limited foci of fibrosis contiguous with damaged renal tubules, whereas more extensive fibrosis is often the result of repeated episodes of superimposed AKI, a phenomenon that has some bearing on the pathogenesis of CKD in humans [58, 59]. Interstitial cellular precursors, such as those of pericytes and fibroblasts, acquire the characteristics of α-smooth muscle actin (α-SMA)-expressing myofibroblasts via PDGFβ-mediated transformation, which contributes to interstitial fibrosis (fig. 5). Loss of endothelial integrity mediated by abnormal VGEF signaling causes 'capillary rarefaction', further impairing tubular regeneration. Failed differentiation of epithelium after AKI leads to deranged gene expression and abnormal signaling, including that involving growth factors, cytokines and autacoids, promoting further pathological changes. Thus, a combination of failed tubular cell differentiation, loss of the microvascular bed with subsequent transmission of high flow and pressure to the glomeruli and proliferation of pro-fibrotic cellular precursors along with activation of mediators of the innate humoral response set the stage for potentially irreversible changes in renal architecture and function [37].

*Role of Hypoxia and Reactive Oxygen Species in the Acute Kidney Injury to Chronic Kidney Disease Transition*
Hypoxia is not only an important mediator of AKI but if persistent also has a role in the pathogenesis of microcirculatory and fibrotic changes that are characteristic of AKI to CKD progression [60, 61]. As explained above, AKI is associated with loss of renal mass, which may lead to a decrease in the volume of the vascular bed [62–64], and hemodynamic abnormalities that result from vasoactive peptides, including activation of the renin-angiotensin system and its inherent pro-fibrotic properties [64]. All of these factors may contribute to

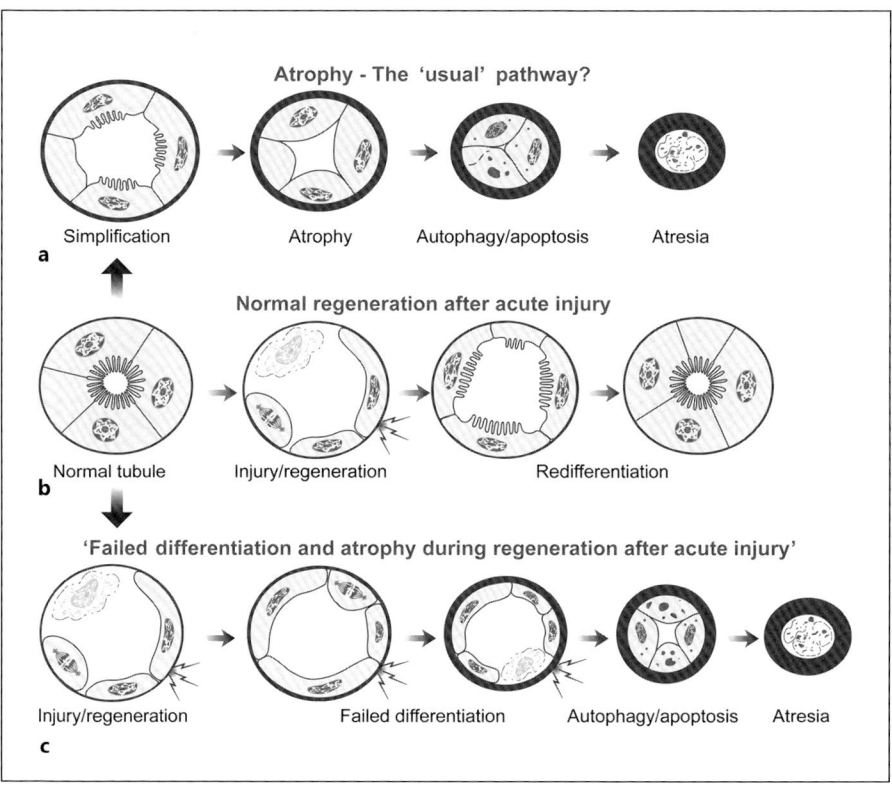

**Fig. 5.** Schematic diagram of the manner by which tubules that are regenerating after acute injury may fail to differentiate and exhibit pro-fibrotic paracrine activity before they become atrophic. **a** The 'usual' pathway of tubule atrophy conceptualized from morphological studies of diseased kidneys involves the simplification of epithelial structure, with progression to autophagy and apoptosis, accompanied by marked thickening of tubule basement membranes. Toward the end of the process, tubules become atretic and enveloped by thick basement membranes or disappear altogether. **b** Normal regeneration of tubules after AKI, with epithelial death, involves initial dedifferentiation, migration, and proliferation of surviving cells, followed by redifferentiation and full restoration of normal structure. Unlike the usual pathway (**a**), tubule cells that survive AKI follow a somewhat different route to become atrophic (**c**). Following dedifferentiation, migration, and proliferation, they fail to redifferentiate. After an indefinite period of time during which they are in a state of 'failed differentiation', these abnormal tubules proceed to develop thick basement membranes and undergo atrophy by autophagy and apoptosis, just as in the usual pathway, and they then disappear by atresia. Hyperactive epithelial paracrine signaling (shown as lightning bolts) in proliferating cells during regeneration becomes suppressed again if tubules redifferentiate normally (**b**) but persists in tubules with a regenerative failed differentiation phenotype (**c**) for an indefinite period of time before atrophy takes place. This paracrine signaling gives rise to inflammation and fibrosis (Reprinted with permission from [37]).

hypoxia-induced tubulo-interstitial fibrosis. Hypoxia-inducible factors (HIFs) play a significant role in the pathophysiology of hypoxia-induced damage. HIFs are transcription factors that regulate the adaptive response against hypoxia and originate in interstitial cells of the kidneys. These adaptations include the transcription of numerous genes involved in angiogenesis, cell proliferation, glucose metabolism, erythropoiesis and apoptosis [61]. HIFs are regulated (inhibited) by a number of prolyl hydroxylases that are predominant in distal convoluted tubules, glomerular podocytes, and interstitial fibroblasts. Pharmacologic or genetic activation of HIFs through inhibition of prolyl hydroxylases holds therapeutic promise in conferring protection after AKI. Using unilateral and bilateral IRI mouse models, Kapitsinou et al. [65] generated HIF-null mice (*HifaHif2a$^{-/-}$* mice) and observed increased injury-associated renal inflammation and fibrosis. Conversely, the use of prolyl hydroxylase inhibitors protected the animals from injury. These effects were mediated by HIF2 but not by HIF1. These findings strongly indicate that full expression of HIF2 after AKI is required to protect animals from the full impact of hypoxic injury.

Renal hypoxia after AKI may be exacerbated by activation of the renin-angiotensin system. Post-AKI rats show an enhanced vasoconstrictor response to ANG II relative to sham-operated controls [66]. IRI also promotes generation of superoxides and other oxygen species, such as hydrogen peroxide and hydroxyl radicals. It has been hypothesized that the link between reactive oxygen species and increased ANG II responsiveness may be relevant to the progression of CKD after AKI through increased fibrosis and altered renal hemodynamics. Thus, male Sprague-Dawley rats were subjected to bilateral IRI or were sham-operated. ANG II infusion significantly decreased renal blood flow (RBF) and increased renal vascular resistance in sham-operated controls, and these changes were even greater in post-IRI animals, who also exhibited a steeper dose-response relationship. Renal oxidative stress was then measured in freshly isolated kidney slices through the oxidation of dihydroethidium. While no dihydroethidium fluorescence was observed in the sham-operated controls, it was consistently present in kidney slices from the post-AKI rats. Most interestingly, at 5 weeks after recovery from AKI, these tissue slices continued to exhibit significantly higher fluorescence than those from the shams. Treatment with apocynin, an inhibitor of NADPH oxidase activity that effectively prevents the production of superoxide ($O_2^-$), significantly reduced the fibrotic effect of ANG II, as revealed by examining the deposition of renal fibroblasts by S100A4 immunohistochemistry. Thus, ANG II and products of reactive oxygen species combine to exacerbate hypoxia and fibrosis during the post-AKI period.

*Role of Biomarkers in Acute Kidney Injury to Chronic Kidney Disease Transition*

Recovery of renal function, as measured by a return of the SC level to baseline or near baseline, after an episode of AKI does not imply that the kidneys have regained the ability to withstand acute changes in RBF or the GFR during a hemodynamic challenge or that they have reacquired intact histological appearances. With the discovery of serum and urinary markers for AKI, recovery or progression has the potential to be accurately assessed in patients with otherwise stable SC levels. In a follow-up study from the Acute Renal Failure Trial Network, investigators examined the predictive levels of a panel of urinary biomarkers, including neutrophil gelatinase-associated lipocalin (NGAL), hepatocyte growth factor (HGF), cystatin C, IL-18, NGAL/matrix metalloproteinase-9, and urinary creatinine. Recovery of renal function was defined as being alive and free of dialysis at 60 days post-hospitalization. Patients who recovered had a higher urinary cystatin level on day 1, a lower urinary HGF level on days 7 and 14 and a decreased urinary NGAL level on day 14. The use of biomarkers combined with the Charlson comorbidity score index was highly predictive of renal recovery (receiver operating characteristic value of 0.94) [67].

**Hypertension Following Acute Kidney Injury**

The development of HTN in humans recovering from an episode of AKI has not been extensively examined. A recent online report by Hsu et al. [68] described 2-year follow-up blood pressure examinations of a cohort of 2,451 patients who experienced AKI and were not known to have HTN prior to the AKI episode. Post-AKI patients had a 22% (95% CI 12–33%) increase in the odds of developing HTN. This finding is not surprising because for several years, studies of animals have clearly linked AKI, with its associated alterations in microvascular function and auto-regulatory properties, with the development of HTN [37, 43]. Pechman et al. [69] studied male Sprague-Dawley rats subjected to IRI and observed a subsequent acute, reversible rise in the SC level. Following a 5-week recovery period, the pressure-natriuresis response was assessed by raising the renal perfusion pressure from 107 to 141 mm Hg. Compared to the controls, the pressure-natriuresis relationship was significantly attenuated in the post-AKI rats. The post-AKI rats also exhibited significant reductions in the GFR and RBF and development of HTN due to increased sodium intake (from a standard 0.4% NaCl diet to a 4% NaCl diet).

## Conclusions

Due to the absence of large prospective clinical trials following patients who have survived a *de novo* episode of AKI to assess their renal outcomes and other complications, our best assessment, based on the large retrospective studies available, is that AKI and CKD are inextricably linked in a bidirectional pathogenetic association that may culminate in the development of late-stage CKD in a large number of patients (fig. 1). The notion that ischemic, toxic or septic insults to the kidneys will for the most part resolve without permanent damage appears obsolete. Even when the SC level returns to baseline, there is considerable basic research and clinical data supporting the notion that an episode of AKI may result in irreversible tubular dropout, interstitial fibrosis and contraction of the vascular bed, limiting the capacity of the kidney to compensate for any further insults that occur. In addition to CKD, an increased death rate and the development of cardiovascular complications, such as heart failure and HTN, may be expected to occur at higher rates in the post-AKI patient population. We propose that most post-AKI patients, especially the elderly and diabetics, should be classified into low- or high-risk groups according to the development of CKD, based in part on existing risk calculators and that when appropriate, they should be entered into a close outpatient follow-up program for the effective management of risk factors for progression to late-stage CKD.

## References

1 Ali T, Khan I, Simpson W, et al: Incidence and outcomes in acute kidney injury: a comprehensive population-based study. J Am Soc Nephrol 2007;18:1292–1298.
2 Saran R, Li Y, Robinson B, et al: US Renal Data System 2014 annual data report: epidemiology of kidney disease in the United States. Am J Kidney Dis 2015;66(suppl 1):S1–S306.
3 Chawla LS, Amdur RL, Shaw A, et al: The Association of Acute Kidney Injury and long-term renal and cardiovascular outcomes in a cohort of US veterans. Clin J Am Soc Nephrol 2014;49:448–456.
4 Wu V-C, Wu C-H, Huang TM, et al: Long-term risk of coronary events after AKI. J Am Soc Nephrol 2014;25:595–605.
5 Lowe KG: The late prognosis in acute tubular necrosis; an interim follow-up report on 14 patients. Lancet 1952;1:1086–1088.
6 Finkenstaedt JT, Merrill JP: Renal function after recovery from renal failure. N Engl J Med 1956;254:1023–1026.
7 Briggs JD, Kennedy AC, Young LN, et al: Renal function after acute tubular necrosis. British Med J 1967;3:513–516.
8 Bonomini V, Stefoni S, Vangelista A: Long-term patient and renal prognosis in acute renal failure. Nephron 1984;36:169–172.
9 Liano F, Felipe C, Tenorio MT, et al: Long-term outcome of acute tubular necrosis: a contribution to its natural history. Kidney Int 2007;71:679–686.

10 James MT, Ghali WA, Tonelli M, et al: Acute kidney injury following coronary angiography is associated with a long-term decline in kidney function. Kidney Int 2010;78:803–809.

11 James MT, Ghali WA, Knudtson ML, et al: Associations between acute kidney injury and cardiovascular and renal outcomes after coronary angiography. Circulation 2011;123: 409–416.

12 Newsome BB, Warnock DG, McClellan WM, et al: Long-term risk of mortality and end-stage renal disease among the elderly after small increases in serum creatinine level during hospitalization for myocardial infarction. Arch Int Med 2008;168:609–616.

13 Wald R, Quinn, RR, Luo J, et al: Chronic dialysis and death among survivors of acute kidney injury requiring dialysis. JAMA 2009; 302:1179–1185.

14 Hsu CY, Chertow GM, McCulloch CE, et al: Nonrecovery of kidney function and death after acute on chronic renal failure. Clin J Am Soc Nephrol 2009;4:891–898.

15 Lafrance JP, Djurdjev O, Levin A: Incidence and outcomes of acute kidney injury in a referred chronic kidney disease cohort. Nephrol Dial Transplant 2010;25:2203–2209.

16 Choi AI, Li Y, Parikh C, et al: Long-term clinical consequences of acute kidney injury in the HIV-infected. Kidney Int 2010;78:478–485.

17 Chertow GM, Burdick E, Honour M, et al: Acute kidney injury, mortality, length of stay, and costs in hospitalized patients. J Am Soc Nephrol 2005;16:3365–3370.

18 Bucaloiu ID, Kirchner HL, Norfolk ER, et al: Increased risk of death and de novo chronic kidney diseases following reversible acute kidney injury. Kidney Int 2012;81:477–485.

19 Amdur RL, Chawla LS, Amodeo S, et al: Outcomes following diagnosis of acute renal failure: focus on acute tubular necrosis. Kidney Int 2009;76:1089–1097.

20 Coca SG, Singanamala S, Parikh CR: Chronic kidney disease after acute kidney injury: a systematic review and meta-analysis. Kidney Int 2012;81:442–448.

21 Lo LJ, Go AS, Chertow GM, et al: Dialysis-requiring acute renal failure increases the risk of progressive chronic kidney disease. Kidney Int 2009;76:893–899.

22 James MT, Hemmelgarn BR, Wiebe N, et al: Glomerular filtration rate, proteinuria, and the incidence and consequences of acute kidney injury: a cohort study. Lancet 2010;376: 2096–2103.

23 Ishani A, Xue JL, Himmelfarb J, et al: Acute kidney injury increases risk of ESRD among elderly. J Am Soc Nephrol 2009;20:223–228.

24 James MT, Grams ME, Woodward M, et al: A meta-analysis of the association of estimated GFR, albuminuria, diabetes mellitus, and hypertension with acute kidney injury. Am J Kidney Dis 2015;66:602–612.

25 Grams ME, Sang Y, Ballew SH, et al: A meta-analysis of the association of estimated GFR, albuminuria, age, race, and sex with acute kidney injury. Am J Kidney Dis 2015;66:591–601.

26 VA/NIH Acute Renal Failure Trial Network, Palevsky PM, Zhang JH, et al. Intensity of renal support in critically ill patients with acute kidney injury. N Engl J Med 2008;359: 7–20.

27 Kidney Diseases/Improving Global Outcomes. KDIGO. Acute Kidney Injury. Kidney International Supplements 2012;2:19–36.

28 Chawla LS, Amdur RL, Amodeo S, et al: The severity of acute kidney injury predicts progression to chronic kidney disease. Kidney Int 2011;79:1361–1369.

29 Perotte A, Ranganath R, Hirsch JS, et al: Risk prediction for chronic kidney disease progression using heterogeneous electronic health record data and time series analysis. J Am Med Inform Assoc 2015;22:872–880.

30 Halbesma N, Jansen DF, Heymans MW, et al: Development and validation of a general population renal risk score. Clin J Am Soc Nephrol 2011;6:1731–1738.

31 Peeters MJ, van Zuilen AD, van den Brand JA, et al: Validation of the kidney failure risk equation in European CKD patients. Nephrol Dial Transplant 2013;28:1773–1779.

32 Herget-Rosenthal S, Dehnen D, Kribben A, et al: Progressive chronic kidney disease in primary care: modifiable risk factors and predictive model. Prev Med 2013;57:357–362.

33 Rucci P, Mandreoli M, Gibertoni D, et al: A clinical stratification tool for chronic kidney disease progression rate based on classification tree analysis. Nephrol Dial Transplant 2014;29:603–610.

34 Kumar S, Liu J, McMahon AP: Defining the acute kidney injury and repair transcriptome. Semin Nephrol 2014;34:404–417.

35 Akcay A, Nguyen Q, Edelstein CL: Mediators of inflammation in acute kidney injury. Mediators Inflamm 2009;2009:137072.

36 Ruggenenti P, Cravedi P, Remuzzi G: Mechanisms and treatment of CKD. J Am Soc Nephrol 2012;23:1917–1928.

37 Venkatachalam MA, Griffin K, Lan R, et al: Acute kidney injury: a springboard for progression in chronic kidney disease. Am J Physiol Renal Physiol 2010;298:F1078–F1094.

38 Sharfuddin AA, Molitoris BA: Pathophysiology of acute kidney injury. Nat Rev Nephrol 2011;7:189–200.

39 Lee SB, Kalluri R: Mechanistic connection between inflammation and fibrosis. Kidney Int Suppl 2010;199:S22–S26.

40 Anders HJ, Schaefer L: Beyond tissue injury-damage-associated molecular patterns, toll-like receptors, and inflammasomes also drive regeneration and fibrosis. J Am Soc Nephrol 2014;25:1387–1400.

41 Duffield JS: Cellular and molecular mechanisms in kidney fibrosis. J Clin Invest 2014; 124:2299–2306.

42 Zager RA: 'Biologic memory' in response to acute kidney injury: cytoresistance, toll-like receptor hyper-responsiveness and the onset of progressive renal disease. Nephrol Dial Transplant 2013;28:1985–1993.

43 Bidani AK, Polichnowski AJ, Loutzenhiser R, et al: Renal microvascular dysfunction, hypertension and CKD progression. Curr Opin Nephrol Hypert 2013;22:1–9.

44 Bonventre JV, Yang L: Cellular pathophysiology of ischemic acute kidney injury. J Clin Invest 2011;121:4210–4221.

45 Emlet DR, Shaw A, Kellum JA: Sepsis-associated AKI: Epithelial cell dysfunction. Semin Nephrol 2015;35:85–95.

46 Basile DP, Fredrich K, Alausa M, et al: Identification of persistently altered gene expression in the kidney after functional recovery from ischemic acute renal failure. Am J Physiol Renal Physiol 2005;288:F953–F963.

47 Basile DP, Martin DR, Hammerman MR: Extracellular matrix-related genes in kidney after ischemic injury: potential role for TGF-β in repair. Am J Physiol 1998;275: F894–F903.

48 Stroo I, Stokman G, Teske GJ, et al: Chemokine expression in renal ischemia/reperfusion injury is most profound during the reparative phase. Int Immunol 2010;22:433–442.

49 Day Y-J, Huang L, Ye H, et al: Renal ischemia-reperfusion injury and adenosine 2A receptors-mediated tissue protection: role of macrophages. Am J Physiol Renal Physiol 2005;288:F722–F731.

50 Tang J, Zhuang S: Epigenetics in acute kidney injury. Curr Opin Nephrol Hypertens 2015; 24:351–358.

51 Rodriguez-Romo R, Berman N, Gomez A, et al: Epigenetic regulation in the acute kidney injury (AKI) to chronic kidney disease transition (CKD). Nephrology (Carlton) DOI: 10.1111/nep.12521.

52 Havasi A, Haegele JA, Gall JM, et al: Histonacetyltransferase (HAT) HBO1 and JADE 1 in epithelial cell regeneration. Am J Pathol 2013; 182:152–162.

53 Bomsztyk K, Flanagin S, Mar D, et al: Synchronous recruitment of epigenetic modifiers to endotoxin synergistically activated TNF-alpha gene in acute kidney injury. PloS One 2013;8:70322.

54 Lorenzen JM, Kaucsar T, Schauerte C, et al: MicroRNA-24 antagonism prevents renal ischemia reperfusion injury. J Am Soc Nephrol 2014;25:2717–2729.

55 Wei Q, Bhatt K, Mi QS, et al: Targeted deletion of Dicer from proximal tubules protects against renal ischemia-reperfusion injury. J Am Soc Nephrol 2010;21:756–761.

56 Ichii O, Otsuka S, Sasaki N, et al: Altered expression of micro-RNA-146a correlates with the development of chronic renal inflammation. Kidney Int 2012;81:280–292.

57 Cantaluppi V, Gatti S, Medica D, et al: Microvesicles derived from endothelial progenitor cells protect the kidney from ischemia-reperfusion injury by microRNA-dependent reprogramming of resident renal cells. Kidney Int 2012;82:412–427.

58 Thakar CV, Christianson A, Himmelfarb J, et al: Acute kidney injury episodes and chronic kidney disease risk in diabetes mellitus. Clin J Am Soc Nephrol 2011;6:2567–2572.

59 Siew ED, Parr SK, Abdel-Khader K, et al: Predictors of recurrent AKI. J Am Soc Nephrol DOI: 10.1681/ASN.2014121218.

60 Tanaka S, Tanaka T, Nangaku M: Hypoxia as a key player in the AKI-CKD transition. Am J Phsyiol Renal Physiol 2014;307:F1187–F1195.

61 Shoji K, Tanaka, T, Nangaku M: Role of hypoxia in progressive chronic kidney disease and implications for therapy. Curr Opin Nephrol Hypertens 2014;23:161–168.

62 Nagasu H, Satoh M, Kidokoro K, et al: Endothelial dysfunction promotes the transition from compensatory renal hypertrophy to kidney injury after unilateral nephrectomy in mice. Am J Physiol Renal Physiol 2012;302: F1402–F1408.

63 Basile DP, Donohoe D, Roethe K, et al: Renal ischemic injury results in permanent damage to peritubular capillaries and influences long term function. Am J Physiol Renal Physiol 2001;281:F887–F899.

64 Basile DP, Friedrich JL, Spahic J, et al: Impaired endothelial proliferation and mesenchymal transition contribute to vascular rarefaction following acute kidney injury. Am J Physiol 2011;300:F721–F733.

65 Kapitsinou PP, Sano H, Michael M, et al: Endothelial HIF-2 mediates protection and recovery from ischemic kidney injury. J Clin Invest 2014;124:2396–2409.

66 Basile DP, Leonard EC, Beal AG, et al: Persistent oxidative stress following renal ischemia-reperfusion injury increases ANG II hemodynamic and fibrotic activity. Am J Physiol Renal Physiol 2012;11:F1494–F1502.

67 Srisawat N, Wen X, Lee M, et al: Urinary biomarkers and renal recovery in critically ill patients with renal support. Clin J Am Soc Nephrol 2011;6:1815–1823.

68 Hsu CY, Hsu RK, Yang J, et al: Elevated BP after AKI. J Am Soc Nephrol DOI: 10.1681/ASN.2014111114.

69 Pechman KR, De Miguel C, Lund H, et al: Recovery form renal ischemia-reperfusion injury is associated with altered renal hemodynamics, blunted pressure natriuresis, and sodium-sensitive hypertension. Am J Physiol Regul Integr Comp Physiol 2009;297:R1358–R1363.

70 Weiss AS, Sandmaier BM, Storer B, et al: Chronic kidney disease following non-myeloablativehematopoietic cell transplantation. Am J Transplant 2006;6:89–94.

71 Ando M, Ohashi K, Akiyama H, et al: Chronic kidney disease in long-term survivors of myeloablative allogeneic hematopoietic cell transplantation; prevalence and risk factors. Nephrol Dial Transplant 2010;25:278–282.

Lakhmir S. Chawla, MD
Medical Service, Department of Veterans Affairs Medical Center
50 Irving Street N.W.
Washington, DC, 20422 (USA)
E-Mail lchawla@ljpc.com

# Electronic Data Systems and Acute Kidney Injury

Wisit Cheungpasitporn[a] · Kianoush Kashani[a,b]

[a]Division of Nephrology and Hypertension and [b]Division of Pulmonary and Critical Care Medicine, Department of Medicine, Mayo Clinic, Rochester, Minn., USA

## Abstract

Acute kidney injury (AKI) is a serious condition that is associated with an increased risk of death, long hospital stays, and high healthcare costs. The best chance of ameliorating the severity of AKI and improving its outcomes is through early recognition and intervention. Electronic health records (EHRs) have now become an integrated part of medical practice in most clinical settings worldwide. Appropriate use of EHRs potentially improves patient care, while poorly designed EHRs could result in unintended consequences. In recent years, EHRs with rule-based algorithms have been used for prompt AKI detection. Although studies using these systems have consistently shown that these EHRs have the capacity to improve the detection of AKI, their application in clinical practice to improve outcomes has shown conflicting results. Future use of EHRs for AKI should go beyond rule-based AKI detection to the creation of AKI-forecasting models for early identification of patients at high risk for AKI and the provision of clinical decision support systems to improve the quality of care and outcomes. Despite significant progress in the field of medical informatics and the growing use of EHRs to enhance the quality of care for AKI patients, these domains remain in the very early stages of development. In this chapter, we review the progress made in this field, as well as the methodologies, applications, and outcomes of using EHRs with AKI alerts. We also discuss the directions that EHR tools need to take to improve the care of patients with AKI.

© 2016 S. Karger AG, Basel

Acute kidney injury (AKI) is a serious condition that affects 7–22% of hospitalized patients and is associated with an increased mortality risk, long hospital stays, increased healthcare expenses and the development of chronic kidney disease [1]. In addition, the incidence of AKI has risen over time due to the increasing number of elderly patients with many comorbidities, the increasing use of potentially nephrotoxic drugs and high-risk interventions, and the use of more sensitive diagnostic criteria. The National Confidential Enquiry into Patient Outcome and Death (NCEPOD) study conducted in the United Kingdom recently reported that 50% of patients who died from AKI received suboptimal care [2].

One of the important steps in improving AKI outcome is early recognition and intervention. Despite the increased awareness of AKI over the last decade, the early detection of AKI remains a challenge. There is a critical need for robust, user-friendly electronic health records (EHRs) with electronic alert capabilities that allow early detection of the condition. The aims of such systems are to automatically and systematically identify all AKI episodes hospital-wide, to notify the designated clinician, and to trigger earlier intervention. In this chapter, we review the progress made in this domain, as well as the methodologies, utilities, and outcomes of using EHRs with electronic AKI alerts. We also discuss the directions that EHR tools need to take to improve the care of patients with AKI.

**Evolution of Electronic Health Records**

Following the implementation of the American Recovery and Reinvestment Act and the Health Information Technology for Economic and Clinical Health Act in 2009, EHR utilization with the explicit purpose of incentivizing providers (e.g., hospitals and physicians) to improve the quality of care has become a nationwide priority [3]. The use of EHRs automates the clinician's workflow and transforms the healthcare system from one that is paper-based to one that utilizes information to support providers in the delivery of a higher quality of care to patients. The EHR systems can maintain complete records of clinical patient encounters. They are also potentially able to support other care-related activities, including evidence-based decision support services, quality management, and outcome reporting [4]. EHRs can incorporate clinically useful tools such as electronic surveillance systems or sniffers, which have been utilized to identify clinical syndromes, including AKI, in a timely and accurate fashion.

In 1966, Weil et al. [5] recorded the first utilization of a digital computer system within intensive care units (ICUs). This report contributed to the birth of the first generation of EHRs, called 'the collectors'. Further inventions associated with information technology and microprocessors subsequently advanced newer generations of EHRs. A summary of EHR generations is shown in table 1. The 3rd generation EHRs has been the most commonly used version at the

**Table 1.** Summary of EHR generations

*First generation (The Collector)*
Simple systems that implement a site-specific solution for the need to obtain clinical data, which is imported through scanning or other forms of collection

*Second generation (The Documenter)*
Basic systems that providers use at the point of care to sufficiently document, rather than solely access, clinical data

*Third generation (The Helper)*
Systems that episodically incorporate and encounter data, use decision support tools for providers, and are functional in both outpatient and inpatient settings at a minimum

*Fourth generation (The Partner)*
Advanced systems that implement additional decision support capabilities, are operational and available across the continuum of care, and provide satisfactory credibility for becoming the patient's legal medical record

*Fifth generation (The Mentor)*
Complex and fully integrated systems that incorporate all previous capabilities and that are a principal source of decision support in guiding patient care for both providers and consumers

bedside as of 1992. This generation has excellent portability and an excellent graphic interface, along with network capabilities. The main issue with the 3rd generation of EHRs is their fragmented nature.

Although the appropriate use of EHRs improves quality of care, poorly designed EHRs could result in harm and unintended consequences, such as increased work tasks associated with computerized order entry; fragmentation of data; loss of communication; and clinical decision support, which may be too rigid, include outdated content, and lead to alert fatigue [6, 7]. In a recent systematic review, Thompson et al. [8] demonstrated a significant decline in in-hospital mortality when electronic surveillance and clinical decision support systems were utilized. However, when other EHR fragments were assessed, the investigators found no improvements in mortality, length of hospital stay or cost.

**Automated Acute Kidney Injury Alerts: Methodologies, Applications, and Outcomes**

In recent years, electronic alert systems have been utilized in the care of AKI patients (table 2). Using rule-based algorithms allows for the classification of patients based on predefined criteria for AKI diagnosis. In the last decade,

**Table 2.** Applications of EHRs in the care of AKI

- Early detection of AKI
- Medication management and dose adjustment
- Identification of high-risk AKI patients
- Enrollment in clinical research trials

precise rules for defining AKI using the RIFLE (risk, injury, failure, loss, end-stage kidney disease), Acute Kidney Injury Network and Kidney Disease: Improving Global Outcomes (KDIGO) criteria have led to improvements in the quality and quantity of research in this field and have enabled investigators to design and test electronic algorithms to detect patients with AKI [9–11].

Electronic alert systems have been developed to fully and/or partially automate the detection of AKI in the hospital setting [12, 13]. Studies using these systems have consistently shown that they have the capacity to improve AKI detection. However, their application in clinical practice produced mixed results. The first reported electronic alert system for AKI was focused on medication management. Rind et al. [14] developed an e-mail alert for patients who were prescribed nephrotoxic or renally excreted medications and developed AKI (defined as an acute increase in the serum creatinine level of >0.5 mg/dl while on nephrotoxic drugs or medications with >50% renal elimination). The investigators found a significant reduction in the dose adjustment time during the intervention period. The risk of significant renal impairment (a twofold increase in the serum creatinine level, to >2.0 mg/dl) was reduced by half. However, the authors were not able to find any impact on mortality or length of hospital stay. McCoy et al. [15] reported a similar system and also designed custom-built AKI alerts within the hospital electronic order entry system. An initial passive signal was sent to the clinician through a computerized order entry system and on printed rounding reports of an acute deterioration in renal function (a rise in the serum creatinine concentration by >0.5 mg/dl over 48 h). This was followed by second and third interruptive alerts requiring physician acknowledgment if the nephrotoxic prescription had not been altered. The AKI alert was linked to recommendations within the medication ordering system that prompted providers to either discontinue or adjust the doses of medications in the presence of reduced kidney function within 24 h of AKI development.

The first hospital-wide electronic warning system created by Thomas et al. [16] generated messages that were sent to the attending physician using a pathology software trigger. In this study, AKI was defined as a >75% rise in serum creatinine. The method identified a group of AKI patients who were at moderate risk of death. However, the accuracy of the tool was limited; two thirds of the patients who subsequently required renal replacement therapy did not generate an alert (either the daily creatinine change was <75% of the previous creatinine level or no previous values were available). The first AKI alert study based on the RIFLE criteria was conducted by Colpaert et al. within a single 56-bed ICU [17]. The study required the manual entry of each baseline creatinine level as well as 2-h data for urine output measurements. When the diagnosis of AKI was met, an automated message was delivered to a real-time digital cordless telephone carried by the care providers. In a follow-up study, investigators reported that AKI alerts increased the timeliness of interventions (mainly fluids or diuretics) but did not improve outcomes [12].

More recently, Selby et al. [18] studied a hospital-wide electronic alert system based on the serum creatinine component of the Acute Kidney Injury Network criteria using the Modified Diet in Renal Disease equation for estimation of baseline serum creatinine. The alert was displayed in the hospital result reporting system alongside creatinine and the estimated glomerular filtration rate. Following the derivation phase of the sniffer, investigators validated the tool and demonstrated a false-positive rate of 1.7% and a false-negative rate of 0.2%.

These observational studies suggest that the use of real-time AKI alerts is feasible and might increase the timeliness of appropriate care. Some studies have also suggested that electronic signals can positively influence physician behavior and improve outcomes [14, 15, 18, 19]. However, a recent single-masked, parallel-group, randomized controlled trial showed no difference in mortality or need for dialysis [13]. In this study, Wilson et al. randomized 2,393 AKI patients into two parallel groups to assess the effect of using a passive, automated, electronic AKI alert system versus usual care on AKI progression, the need for dialysis and death. Patients were assigned to receive either usual care or AKI alerts and were stratified by surgical versus medical admission and by ICU versus non-ICU location. The care providers and the unit pharmacists were alerted to the presence of AKI via a page sent to their mobile phones. The alerts directed the clinicians to a link that provided best practice guidelines. The alerts were sent within 1 h of reporting of the serum creatinine level. To avoid alert fatigue, the alert was only sent once for each episode of AKI. The investigators found no effect on AKI progression, the need for dialysis or death. The intervention also showed no impact on the process of care, such as the utilization of a fluid bolus or medication modification. The authors noted that the intervention group in the surgical ward had higher rates of nephrology consultations (12 vs. 5%) and initiation of dialysis (6 vs. 3%).

**Table 3.** NHS automated AKI algorithm

| AKI criteria | Definition for AKI (one of the three) |
|---|---|
| Criterion 1 | Serum creatinine ≥1.5 times higher than the median of all creatinine 8–365 days ago |
| Criterion 2 | Serum creatinine ≥1.5 times greater than the lowest creatinine within 7 days |
| Criterion 3 | Serum creatinine >26 µmol/l (0.3 mg/dl) higher than the minimum creatinine within 48 h |

| AKI stage | Classification requirements |
|---|---|
| Stage 1 | Rise in creatinine of >26 µmol/l or index/reference ≥1.5 and <2 |
| Stage 2 | Index/reference ≥2 and <3 |
| Stage 3 | Index/reference ≥3 or ≥1.5 and index creatinine >354 µmol/l (4 mg/dl, or three times the upper reference interval if age <18) |

AKI can be diagnosed if one of the three criteria is met. Staging is based on a comparison of serum creatinine (index) with a reference test. When a creatinine level is outside of the reference range but a previous creatinine measurement from within 1 year is unavailable, the test is 'flagged' as abnormal (with chronicity uncertain).

Although the results were discouraging for the use of rule-based electronic surveillance tools, the study limitations made it difficult to dismiss the potential role of these devices in the care of patients with AKI. The expected value of using automated surveillance tools for the detection of AKI is to identify AKI earlier, so that clinicians can provide such patients with appropriate preventive and/or potential therapeutic measures. In the above-mentioned study, a urine output criterion was not used. Urine output is a more sensitive and earlier marker of AKI, particularly in the hospital floor setting, where the frequency of serum creatinine measurement is not high and the use of a regular urine output criterion could lead to an earlier diagnosis of AKI. Additionally, the investigators did not provide any information regarding the validity and reliability of their tool. The passive nature of the alert, which did not need any acknowledgment from the clinicians, is another limitation of the study. Both the AKI alert and the usual-care groups received their care in the same hospital departments, which may have resulted in cross-contamination (Hawthorne effect).

In 2014, the National Health System (NHS) in the United Kingdom developed a mandatory national automated algorithm for detecting AKI based on the KDIGO definition. The NHS algorithm requires that one of the three criteria that are outlined in table 3 is satisfied. Sawhney et al. [20] enrolled 127,851 patients from the United Kingdom's NHS. The three criteria used for the NHS algorithm were found to be more sensitive for detecting AKI according to the

International Classification of Diseases, 10th Revision, when compared with the algorithm used by Wilson et al. [13]. In this study, >91% of patients who were ultimately identified as having AKI based on the International Classification of Diseases, 10th Revision, had a positive alert. In comparison, the sensitivity of the warning system was only 74.2% in the trial by Wilson et al. In addition, most of the alerts occurred >2 days following admission, despite the fact that the majority of AKIs occur at the time of admission or within 2 days following admission [21]. Delayed alerting may therefore have mitigated the outcome benefits of using such an alert system.

*Challenges with Using Serum Creatinine and Urine Output Criteria*
The KDIGO criteria for the definition of AKI require that absolute or relative changes in serum creatinine levels be determined within 48 h and 7 days, respectively. Therefore, to define AKI, knowing the baseline serum creatinine is critical; however, there is no consensus on how to optimally determine baseline serum creatinine. A lack of access to the baseline serum creatinine level in the clinical setting is very common. Imputation of missing results by backward calculation using the Modified Diet in Renal Disease formula, assuming an estimated glomerular filtration rate of 75 ml/min/1.73 m$^2$, has been proposed as an alternative for those who have not undergone serum creatinine measurement within the 7–365 days prior to their admission [22]. The other challenge in defining AKI using the KDIGO criteria is the accurate collection and timely documentation of urine output. Therefore, most studies on AKI alerts have used only the serum creatinine criterion, rather than both criteria [16, 18]. In a recent study by Ahmed et al., both criteria were used to identify AKI, with a specificity of 96% and sensitivity of 88% [23].

*Sensitivity, Specificity, and Context Recognition of Acute Kidney Injury Sniffers*
To maximize the clinical benefit of using an AKI sniffer, apart from the high sensitivity and specificity of the associated algorithms, it must be able to monitor care provider behaviors as well. If an AKI sniffer correctly identifies the syndrome and detects suboptimal care, then it should promptly alert clinicians. This alert would be very meaningful and may potentially advance patient care. In contrast, if the sniffer generated many false-positive alerts or ignores optimized care provided to true-positive AKI patients, it would only serve as a distractor. To avoid distraction, the first step is to define the algorithms with high sensitivity and specificity. Then, a smart sniffer should alarm clinicians only when the best care for the management of AKI is not provided.

In addition, sniffers that are utilized to identify patients who need more costly interventions with potentially higher complication rates should be significantly more specific than sniffers that are used to screen ICUs for administrative purposes.

*Risk Stratification for Acute Kidney Injury*

In the past few decades, statistical models that predict adverse outcomes have been widely used to improve the quality of care, to risk-stratify patients and to provide individual prognostications [24, 25]. Several risk stratification and forecasting models have been developed to predict AKI following specific coronary arterial bypass grafting surgery and percutaneous coronary interventions and contrast-induced AKI using clinical registry data [26–28]. While most of these models perform well, they have not been broadly utilized at the bedside due to challenges in the real-time bedside calculation and analysis of scores. Using EHRs and electronic algorithms to utilize these models is feasible and may potentially improve the quality of care for AKI patients. Matheny et al. [29] used structured clinical data collected from EHRs and constructed risk stratification models to predict AKI with an area under the receiver operating characteristic curve of 0.78. Future work in this field will include efforts to enhance model performance by incorporating bar-coded medication dosing and administration data as well as implementing these models in clinical decision support systems and prospectively assessing their utility.

There are two different types of forecasting models for hospitalized patients. Static forecasting models are created once, at a single point in time, using the actual value for each subsequent forecast assigned to each patient, which would be directly correlated with the risk of AKI development in the future. In contrast, dynamic prediction models incorporate parameters such as baselines and physiologic, hemodynamic, pharmacologic and pathophysiologic variables that are frequently adjusted when new information becomes available. Dynamic models are potentially more valid, particularly for entities that have dynamic or evolutionary behaviors. Accurate and real-time AKI forecasting enables appropriate resource allocation, earlier intervention, and dynamic updated risk estimation based on a patient's health status assessment and exposure to anticipated clinical interventions.

*Electronic Health Records as a Research Tool*

Patient enrollment in AKI-related time-sensitive studies, particularly in the critical care field, can be cumbersome and expensive. Coordinators need to screen EHRs for eligibility or rely on notifications from bedside providers. Utilizing

EHRs with electronic alerts to identify patients who meet study criteria could potentially decrease the cost of a study. Future EHRs should support the identification and recognition of patients with potential or established critical illness outside of critical care areas for the purposes of timely clinical intervention and enrollment in clinical research trials.

*Future Role of Electronic Health Records in Acute Kidney Injury*

In the future, the development of more sophisticated EHRs not only should enable the detection of AKI but also should be extended to the development of algorithm-based predictive, diagnostic, and risk stratification instruments. In the randomized controlled trial conducted by Wilson et al. [13], given the absence of any detectable differences in provider behavior, the finding that AKI alerts did not improve clinical outcomes is not unexpected. The alert prompted providers to visit a website for more information on AKI, but no data were given on whether traffic to this site was increased as a result. Conversely, making patient-specific recommendations lends itself to better physician acceptance and possibly better patient outcomes. Holding AKI alert systems to the standard of improving outcomes will require the coupling of better therapies to these systems. In the future, real-time EHRs should deliver decision support, care bundles, and management recommendations within the clinical workflow at the time and location of decision making. Additionally, future EHRs should recognize clinical contexts, patient characteristics, and patient exposures (e.g., nephrotoxic drugs, sepsis). Such instruments could aid in the identification of patients who are at the highest risk and will benefit from targeted, disease-specific interventions.

Even if alerts offer lead time, the time that they provide may not be sufficient, and kidney injury may already be irreversible. The use of urine output or novel biomarkers [30] in combination with EHRs may change this paradigm. Moreover, any future EHRs should support the identification of patients with potential or established critical illnesses outside of critical care areas for the purpose of timely clinical intervention and enrollment in clinical trials.

In summary, notwithstanding the significant advances in the use of EHRs to better the quality of care of AKI patients, these fields remain in the very beginning steps of evolution. There are real benefits to be gained from using an AKI alert system. The spectrum of electronic warning system benefits could range from the early and precise detection of AKI to the accurate prediction of this syndrome, supplemented with clinical decision support systems for higher-risk patients. Future progress and research in this field would open new horizons for exploration within the field.

## References

1 Susantitaphong P, et al: World incidence of AKI: a meta-analysis. Clin J Am Soc Nephrol: CJASN 2013;8:1482–1493.
2 National Confidential Enquiry into Patient Outcome and Death: Adding Insult to Injury: A Review of the Care of Patients who Died in Hospital with a Primary Diagnosis of Acute Kidney Injury (Acute Renal Failure). London, The National Confidential Enquiry Into Patient Outcome and Death, 2009.
3 Lenert L, Sundwall DN: Public health surveillance and meaningful use regulations: a crisis of opportunity. Am J Public Health 2012;102: e1–e7.
4 National Institutes of Health, National Center for Research Resources, Electronic Health Records Overview; in McLean VA (ed): Center for Enterprise Modernization. MITRE Corporation, 2006.
5 Weil MH, Shubin H, Rand W: Experience with a digital computer for study and improved management of the critically ill. JAMA 1966;198:1011–1016.
6 Kashani K, Herasevich V: Sniffing out acute kidney injury in the ICU: do we have the tools? Curr Opin Crit Care 2013;19:531–536.
7 Han YY, et al: Unexpected increased mortality after implementation of a commercially sold computerized physician order entry system. Pediatrics 2005;116:1506–1512.
8 Thompson G, et al: Impact of the electronic medical record on mortality, length of stay, and cost in the hospital and ICU: a systematic review and metaanalysis. Crit Care Med 2015;43:1276–1282.
9 Bellomo R, et al: Acute renal failure – definition, outcome measures, animal models, fluid therapy and information technology needs: the Second International Consensus Conference of the Acute Dialysis Quality Initiative (ADQI) Group. Crit Care 2004;8:R204–R212.
10 Mehta RL, et al: Acute Kidney Injury Network: report of an initiative to improve outcomes in acute kidney injury. Crit Care 2007; 11:R31.
11 Kidney Disease: Improving Global Outcomes (KDIGO): KDIGO Clinical Practice Guidelines for Acute Kidney Injury. Kid Int Suppl 2012;2:1–138.
12 Colpaert K, et al: Impact of real-time electronic alerting of acute kidney injury on therapeutic intervention and progression of RIFLE class. Crit Care Med 2012;40:1164–1170.
13 Wilson FP, et al: Automated, electronic alerts for acute kidney injury: a single-blind, parallel-group, randomised controlled trial. Lancet 2015;385:1966–1974.
14 Rind DM, et al: Effect of computer-based alerts on the treatment and outcomes of hospitalized patients. Arch Intern Med 1994;154: 1511–1517.
15 McCoy AB, et al: A computerized provider order entry intervention for medication safety during acute kidney injury: a quality improvement report. Am J Kidney Dis 2010;56: 832–841.
16 Thomas M, Sitch A, Dowswell G: The initial development and assessment of an automatic alert warning of acute kidney injury. Nephrol Dial Transplant 2011;26:2161–2168.
17 Colpaert K, et al: Implementation of a real-time electronic alert based on the RIFLE criteria for acute kidney injury in ICU patients. Acta Clin Belg Suppl 2007;62(suppl 2):322–325.
18 Selby NM, et al: Use of electronic results reporting to diagnose and monitor AKI in hospitalized patients. Clin J Am Soc Nephrol: CJASN 2012;7:533–540.
19 Colpaert K, et al: Implementation of a real-time electronic alert based on the RIFLE criteria for acute kidney injury in ICU patients. Acta Clinica Belgica. Supplementum 2007;62: 322–325.
20 Sawhney S, et al: Acute kidney injury-how does automated detection perform? Nephrol Dial Transplant 2015;30:1853–1861.
21 Wonnacott A, et al: Epidemiology and outcomes in community-acquired versus hospital-acquired AKI. Clin J Am Soc Nephrol: CJASN 2014;9:1007–1014.
22 Ahmed S, et al: Population-based estimated reference creatinine values: a novel method of a robust electronic acute kidney injury alert system. Nephron Clin Pract 2014;128: 166–170.
23 Ahmed A, et al: Development and validation of electronic surveillance tool for acute kidney injury: A retrospective analysis. J Crit Care 2015(0).

24 Hunt JP, Meyer AA: Predicting survival in the intensive care unit. Curr Probl Surg 1997; 34:527–599.
25 Randolph AG, Guyatt GH, Carlet J: Understanding articles comparing outcomes among intensive care units to rate quality of care. Evidence Based Medicine in Critical Care Group. Crit Care Med 1998;26:773–781.
26 Mehran R, et al: A simple risk score for prediction of contrast-induced nephropathy after percutaneous coronary intervention: development and initial validation. J Am Coll Cardiol 2004;44:1393–1399.
27 Thakar CV, et al: A clinical score to predict acute renal failure after cardiac surgery. J Am Soc Nephrol 2005;16:162–168.
28 Wijeysundera DN, et al: Derivation and validation of a simplified predictive index for renal replacement therapy after cardiac surgery. JAMA 2007;297:1801–1809.
29 Matheny ME, et al: Development of inpatient risk stratification models of acute kidney injury for use in electronic health records. Med Decis Making 2010;30:639–650.
30 Kashani K, Kellum JA: Novel biomarkers indicating repair or progression after acute kidney injury. Curr Opin Nephrol Hypertens 2015;24:21–27.

Kianoush Kashani, MD
Mayo Clinic
200 First Street SW
Rochester, MN 55905 (USA)
E-Mail kashani.kianoush@mayo.edu

# Fluid Management in Acute Kidney Injury

Chiao-Lin Chuang

Division of General Medicine, Department of Medicine, Taipei Veterans General Hospital, and Department of Medicine, National Yang-Ming University School of Medicine, Taipei, Taiwan

## Abstract

The goal of fluid therapy in critical care medicine is to restore hemodynamic stability and vital organ perfusion while avoiding interstitial edema. Acute kidney injury (AKI) is a common complication in critically ill patients. Decisions regarding fluid management in critically ill patients with AKI are difficult, as these patients often have accompanying oliguria as well as body fluid overload. Both hypovolemia and volume overload are associated with increased morbidity and mortality in critical care patients; therefore, accurate assessment of the intravascular volume status as well as the response to fluid replacement remains one of the most challenging and important issues for clinicians in daily practice. Newer dynamic preload indexes, such as stroke volume variation and pulse pressure variation in conjunction with the end-expiratory occlusion test and the passive leg-raising test, have been shown to be more reliable indicators for accurate evaluation of fluid responsiveness in critically ill patients than static pressure measurements, such as central vein pressure and pulmonary artery occlusion pressure. In patients with established AKI who are unresponsive to fluid administration, fluid restriction is the treatment of choice. When fluid therapy is indicated for AKI patients, isotonic crystalloids should be the preferred agents in the absence of hemorrhagic shock. Balanced solutions may reduce the risk of hyperchloremic acidosis and kidney injury. In summary, volume management is an integral part of the care of critically ill patients with AKI. An optimal strategy might involve a timely period of guided fluid resuscitation with appropriate solutions, followed by an appropriate fluid balance.

© 2016 S. Karger AG, Basel

Acute kidney injury (AKI) is a frequent, life-threatening complication in critically ill patients. The Beginning and Ending Supportive Therapy for the Kidney (BEST Kidney) study investigators revealed the fact that septic shock is the most common factor contributing to AKI in intensive care units (ICUs), accounting for 47.5% of AKI patients [1]. Due to a lack of effective pharmacotherapies, treatment aimed at reversing or preventing septic AKI remains primarily based on supportive hemodynamic management. As a result, intravenous fluids play a critical role in the resuscitation of critically ill patients with severe sepsis or septic shock [2, 3]. From a renal perspective, the expected physiologic benefit of fluid resuscitation is based on the improvement of renal blood flow (RBF) and renal perfusion pressure resulting from restoration of effective circulating volume. However, AKI appears to be irreversible after achieving a supra-normal cardiac index, despite the fact that renal hypoperfusion is believed to contribute to the development of sepsis-induced renal dysfunction [4]. Significant changes in stroke volume (SV) and mean arterial pressure (MAP) induced by fluid challenge did not improve renal perfusion in patients with AKI [5]. Furthermore, septic patients with AKI often present with accompanying oliguria as well as body fluid overload, which is associated with increased capillary permeability as well as interstitial and cellular edema. Since the kidney is an encapsulated organ, fluid accumulation related to tissue edema would lead to a decrease in RBF and the glomerular filtration rate. Fluid overload in critically ill patients may also predispose them to the development of intra-abdominal hypertension, which is an additional risk factor for AKI [6]. In this regard, fluid overload is both a consequence of and a causative factor for AKI in critically ill patients. Overzealous fluid resuscitation and the resultant positive fluid balance in AKI are associated with increased lengths of ICU and hospital stays, a higher risk of renal nonrecovery and mortality [7–9]. A subgroup analysis of patients who developed AKI in the Fluid and Catheter Treatment Trial (FACTT) showed that a positive fluid balance after AKI carried a 'dose effect' association with the risk of death, with approximately 1.6-fold higher risk per liter/day of fluid accumulated [10]. Therefore, an optimal strategy and optimal target endpoints for fluid therapy during the resuscitation of critically ill patients with AKI are extremely imperative. A number of randomized control studies that provide evolutionary knowledge regarding the timing, the dose, and the type of fluid management used for the treatment of critically ill patients have been published during the past decades.

**Type of Fluid Therapy**

*Crystalloids or Colloids*
The physiologic rationale for administering colloids during resuscitation is to expand the plasma volume more effectively. The large-molecular-weight

solutes present in colloid solutions are theoretically resistant to passing through capillary membranes and hence preserve intravascular oncotic pressure and prevent fluid extravasation. However, the advantages of colloids have been questioned for years. The Saline versus Albumin Fluid Evaluation (SAFE) study, a landmark study comparing the effects of 4% albumin versus normal saline in 6,997 critically ill patients, found no difference in all-cause mortality at 28 days [11]. In addition, subgroup analysis revealed an association of albumin with higher mortality in patients with traumatic brain injury [12]. Similarly, the Albumin Italian Outcome Sepsis (ALBIOS) trial, which compared 20% albumin to crystalloid in septic patient resuscitation, showed no survival benefit [13]. These results may be accounted for by the fact that the vascular endothelium is disrupted in critically ill patients. In the setting of increased capillary permeability with extravasation of proteins into the extracellular space, colloids may worsen edema by increasing interstitial oncotic pressure and fluid accumulation, resulting in further impediment of tissue perfusion.

Recently, the clinical association of synthetic colloid use with renal dysfunction has been confirmed by several clinical trials. The Scandinavian Starch for Severe Sepsis/Septic Shock Trial (6S) [14] and the Crystalloid versus Hydroxyethyl Starch Trial (CHEST) [15] reported a significantly higher risk of AKI or requirement of renal replacement therapy in patients receiving fluid resuscitation with hydroxyethyl starch compared with crystalloid solutions. Several hypotheses have been formulated to explain AKI following colloid administration, including the accumulation of low-molecular-weight fractions in renal tubules and osmotic nephrosis [16]. Given the evidence of the lack of significant clinical benefit from and the potential harmful effects of colloids, the current consensus statement of the Kidney Disease: Improving Global Outcomes clinical practice guidelines suggests that isotonic crystalloids, rather than colloids (albumin or hydroxyethyl starch), be used as initial management for the expansion of intravascular volume in patients at risk for AKI or with AKI in the absence of hemorrhagic shock [17].

*Are All Crystalloids the Same?*
The most commonly used crystalloid in clinical practice is 0.9% saline with supra-physiologic levels of sodium and chloride. Resuscitation with moderate-to-large amounts of 0.9% saline induces hyperchloremia and metabolic acidosis [18], which has been associated with a decline in RBF in an animal study [19] and in healthy human volunteers [20]. Based on a study on 22,851 surgical patients with normal preoperative serum chloride concentrations and renal function, patients with postoperative hyperchloremia were more likely to

**Table 1.** Compositions of human plasma and commonly used solutions

|  | Human plasma | Colloid | | Crystalloid | | | | |
| --- | --- | --- | --- | --- | --- | --- | --- | --- |
|  |  | 4% albumin | 6% HES | 0.9% NaCl | balanced | | | |
|  |  |  |  |  | Ringer's lactate | PlasmaLyte 148 | Hartmann's solution | |
| Sodium, mmol/l | 140 | 140 | 154 | 154 | 130 | 140 | 129 |
| Chloride, mmol/l | 100 | 128 | 154 | 154 | 109 | 98 | 109 |
| Potassium, mmol/l | 4.5 | 0 | 0 | 0 | 4 | 5 | 5 |
| Calcium, mmol/l | 2.5 | 0 | 0 | 0 | 2 | 0 | 2 |
| Magnesium, mmol/l | 1 | 0 | 0 | 0 | 0 | 1.5 | 0 |
| Bicarbonate, mmol/l | 25 | 0 | 0 | 0 | 0 | 0 | 0 |
| Acetate, mmol/l | 0 | 0 | 0 | 0 | 0 | 27 | 0 |
| Lactate, mmol/l | 0 | 0 | 0 | 0 | 28 | 0 | 29 |
| Gluconate, mmol/l | 0 | 0 | 0 | 0 | 0 | 23 | 0 |
| Octanoate, mmol/l | 0 | 6.4 | 0 | 0 | 0 | 0 | 0 |

develop postoperative renal dysfunction [21]. In this regard, current studies have largely focused on comparing the effects of different crystalloids. The ideal electrolyte solution may be one that reasonably parallels the plasma (table 1). Balanced fluids, such as lactate Ringer's, Hartmann's solution, and PlasmaLyte, have an electrolyte composition close to that of human plasma. The use of these chloride-restrictive fluids for volume resuscitation has been associated with significantly lower in-hospital mortality [22], a decreased incidence of AKI and the need for renal replacement therapy in ICUs [23]. More large-scale randomized control trials will be required to support the renal protectiveness of balanced solutions in the treatment of critically ill patients at risk for AKI or with AKI.

## Timing of Fluid Management

*Rationale for Fluid Replacement in Acute Kidney Injury*
According to this conceptual framework, AKI in critical illness is believed to be the consequence of reduced cardiac output (CO) and systemic hypotension, leading to a decrease in renal perfusion and the glomerular filtration rate. Thus, the resuscitation of patients in shock needs to be timely and adequate to prevent or attenuate AKI. For years, early goal-directed therapy (EGDT), aiming to optimize tissue oxygen transport by continuous monitoring of MAP, central venous pressure (CVP), and central venous oxygen saturation, has been regarded as standard of care and incorporated into the Surviving Sepsis guidelines [3].

However, the study by Rivers et al. did not show evidence of renal protection from EGDT [2]. In addition, the survival benefit was not replicated in any of the recently published 3 large multicenter randomized controlled studies examining the effect of EGDT in sepsis (the Protocolized Care for Early Septic Shock (ProCESS) trial, the Australasian Resuscitation in Sepsis Evaluation (ARISE) trial, and the Protocolised Management in Sepsis (ProMISe) trial) [24–26], although their study designs were quite similar. Not surprisingly, there were no significant differences in the incidence of AKI or the use of renal replacement therapy, irrespective of the treatment approach used for severe sepsis. These results challenge our understanding of the potential benefits of early fluid resuscitation in septic shock.

The key point is probably not just the amount of fluid resuscitation but also mostly the achievement of hemodynamic optimization with that volume. The expected hemodynamic benefit of volume expansion is an increase in SV and subsequent improvement of organ perfusion. Only patients who show a significant increase in SV following a fluid challenge are considered to benefit, suggesting that they are fluid responders. If this is not the case, volume expansion may only exert adverse effects, without any hemodynamic benefit. Therefore, it is crucial to determine whether a patient is fluid responsive or not during resuscitation. This begets the question of what the exact target of fluid therapy is.

*How Can Fluid Responsiveness Be Measured in Critically Ill Patients?*
Traditional assessment of fluid status depends on physical examination accompanied by chest X-ray, which provides limited value in critically ill patients. Static cardiac filling pressure, such as CVP and pulmonary artery occlusion pressure, is therefore widely used to assess the volume status and fluid responsiveness in ICUs. However, cumulative evidence from clinical studies has clearly shown that using MAP [27], CVP [28], and pulmonary artery occlusion pressure [29] to guide fluid management has poor predictive value. The weak relationship between traditional indicators and volume responsiveness suggests a need for better parameters to discriminate fluid responders from nonresponders among critically ill patients.

Fluid is usually administered based on the expectation of increasing cardiac preload and SV. The Frank-Starling curve is commonly used to define the relationship between ventricular preload and SV. An increase in preload with volume challenge will induce a significant increase in SV only if the ventricle operates on the steeper ascending portion of the curve, which is suggestive of preload dependence and fluid responsiveness. Based on the curvilinear relationship, the SV will proportionately increase with increasing preload until it reaches the

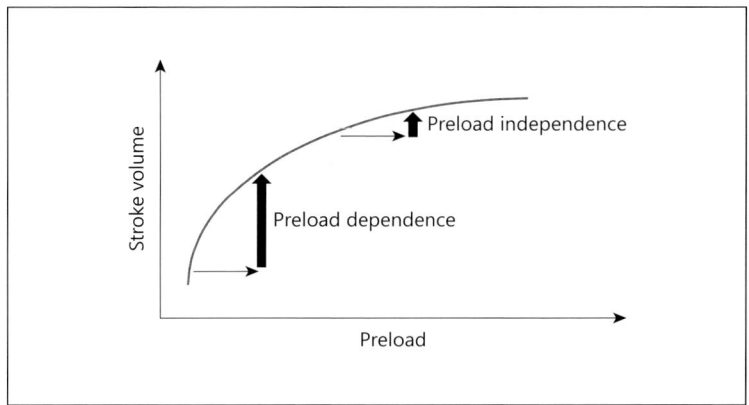

**Fig. 1.** Stroke volume variation is a dynamic indicator of fluid response. The same increase in preload results in significantly different changes in stroke volume depending on the position on the Frank-Starling curve. An increase in preload with volume challenge will induce a higher increase in stroke volume only if the ventricle operates on the steeper ascending portion of the curve, which is suggestive of preload dependence and fluid responsiveness.

plateau of the curve, which is suggestive of fluid nonresponsiveness (fig. 1). This dynamic concept is further applied to measure the variations in SV induced by positive-pressure ventilation.

*How Can Fluid Responsiveness Be Predicted in Critically Ill Patients?*
To test fluid responsiveness, a change in preload must be provoked while monitoring the subsequent change in SV. Since classic fluid challenge may be irreversible and lead to fluid overload, particularly in AKI patients, several tests have been developed to detect volume responsiveness before administering fluid in recent years. For mechanically ventilated patients, positive pressure mechanical ventilation induces a reduction in left ventricular preload through a decrease in venous return. Therefore, stroke volume variation (SVV) induced by mechanical ventilation will be higher when a patient is a fluid responder. Numerous clinical studies have consistently confirmed the excellent value of respiratory variation in SV or in surrogates for predicting fluid responsiveness [30, 31]. SVV and pulse pressure variation (PPV) are the two most commonly used methods. Nowadays, there are a variety of commercially available minimally invasive monitoring devices that utilize pulse contour analysis to provide automated calculations of CO as well as dynamic measures of preload responsiveness. However, the presence of arrhythmias and spontaneous breathing activity may preclude these indices from being used.

The end-expiratory occlusion (EEO) test is another preload challenge based on heart-lung interactions that can be used to predict fluid responsiveness in ventilated patients. This test is performed by briefly interrupting ventilation at end expiration to increase venous return and CO in fluid responders [32]. The EEO test is reliable in patients with arrhythmia or acute respiratory distress syndrome (low tidal volume and low lung compliance), a condition where PPV and SVV may be unreliable. To assess fluid responsiveness in patients with spontaneous breathing activity, the passive leg-raising test, a reversible maneuver that mimics rapid volume challenge by shifting venous blood from the lower limbs toward the cardiac chambers, has been well validated as a reliable index of fluid responsiveness [33].

In addition, echocardiography, a noninvasive bedside procedure for the measurement of dynamic changes in the diameters of the inferior vena cava (IVC) and superior vena cava (SVC), allows for accurate assessment of fluid responsiveness during spontaneous breathing and mechanical ventilation [34, 35].

## Conclusion

The cornerstone of volume management in critically ill patients with AKI is to maintain an effective circulating volume and tissue oxygenation while avoiding interstitial and tissue edema. Thus, fluid responsiveness should be detected before volume expansion. Accounting for the relationship between fluid challenge and SV, the physiologic concept of preload dependence is of great value in guiding fluid therapy in critical care. The analysis of mechanical ventilation-induced variation in preload to track changes in SV and PPV as well as the IVC and SVC diameters has shown promise in numerous studies. Both the EEO test and the passive leg-raising test can be used as alternative methods of preload challenge to determine fluid responsiveness in cases of spontaneous breathing activity and/or cardiac arrhythmias. When fluid therapy is indicated for AKI patients, isotonic crystalloids, and particularly balanced solutions, should be the preferred agents in patients at risk for AKI or with AKI. Finally, it is essential to emphasize that individualized fluid strategies should be considered in the setting of a heterogeneous patient population with complex clinical conditions. In summary, although the consensus remains elusive, goal-directed fluid therapy based on a patient's underlying pathophysiology that is guided by dynamic preload parameters (e.g., PPV, SVV, and dynamic changes in the IVC and SVC diameters) to ensure the hemodynamic optimization represents an ideal approach in critical care.

## References

1 Uchino S, Kellum JA, Bellomo R, Doig GS, Morimatsu H, Morgera S, Schetz M, Tan I, Bouman C, Macedo E, Gibney N, Tolwani A, Ronco C, Beginning and Ending Supportive Therapy for the Kidney (BEST Kidney) Investigators: Acute renal failure in critically ill patients: a multinational, multicenter study. JAMA 2005;294:813–818.

2 Rivers E, Nguyen B, Havstad S, Ressler J, Muzzin A, Knoblich B, Peterson E, Tomlanovich M, Early Goal-Directed Therapy Collaborative Group: Early goal-directed therapy in the treatment of severe sepsis and septic shock. N Engl J Med 2001;345:1368–1377.

3 Dellinger RP, Levy MM, Rhodes A, Annane D, Gerlach H, Opal SM, Sevransky JE, Sprung CL, Douglas IS, Jaeschke R, Osborn TM, Nunnally ME, Townsend SR, Reinhart K, Kleinpell RM, Angus DC, Deutschman CS, Machado FR, Rubenfeld GD, Webb SA, Beale RJ, Vincent JL, Moreno R, Surviving Sepsis Campaign Guidelines Committee including the Pediatric Subgroup: Surviving sepsis campaign: international guidelines for management of severe sepsis and septic shock: 2012. Crit Care Med 2013;41:580–637.

4 Gattinoni L, Brazzi L, Pelosi P, Latini R, Tognoni G, Pesenti A, Fumagalli R: A trial of goal-oriented hemodynamic therapy in critically ill patients. SvO2 Collaborative Group. N Engl J Med 1995;333:1025–1032.

5 Schnell D, Camous L, Guyomarc'h S, Duranteau J, Canet E, Gery P, Dumenil AS, Zeni F, Azoulay E, Darmon M: Renal perfusion assessment by renal Doppler during fluid challenge in sepsis. Crit Care Med 2013;41:1214–1220.

6 Dalfino L, Tullo L, Donadio I, Malcangi V, Brienza N: Intra-abdominal hypertension and acute renal failure in critically ill patients. Intensive Care Med 2008;34:707–713.

7 Payen D, de Pont AC, Sakr Y, Spies C, Reinhart K, Vincent JL, Sepsis Occurrence in Acutely Ill Patients (SOAP) Investigators: A positive fluid balance is associated with a worse outcome in patients with acute renal failure. Crit Care 2008;12:R74.

8 Grams ME, Estrella MM, Coresh J, Brower RG, Liu KD, National Heart, Lung, and Blood Institute Acute Respiratory Distress Syndrome Network: Fluid balance, diuretic use, and mortality in acute kidney injury. Clin J Am Soc Nephrol 2011;6:966–973.

9 Teixeira C, Garzotto F, Piccinni P, Brienza N, Iannuzzi M, Gramaticopolo S, Forfori F, Pelaia P, Rocco M, Ronco C, Anello CB, Bove T, Carlini M, Michetti V, Cruz DN; NEFROlogia e Cura INTensiva (NEFROINT) investigators: Fluid balance and urine volume are independent predictors of mortality in acute kidney injury. Crit Care 2013;17:R14.

10 Bouchard J, Soroko SB, Chertow GM, Himmelfarb J, Ikizler TA, Paganini EP, Mehta RL, Program to Improve Care in Acute Renal Disease (PICARD) Study Group: Fluid accumulation, survival and recovery of kidney function in critically ill patients with acute kidney injury. Kidney Int 2009;76:422–427.

11 Finfer S, Bellomo R, Boyce N, French J, Myburgh J, Norton R, SAFE Study Investigators: A comparison of albumin and saline for fluid resuscitation in the intensive care unit. N Engl J Med 2004;350:2247–2256.

12 Myburgh J, Cooper DJ, Finfer S, Bellomo R, Norton R, Bishop N, Kai Lo S, Vallance S: Saline or albumin for fluid resuscitation in patients with traumatic brain injury. N Engl J Med 2007;357:874–884.

13 Caironi P, Tognoni G, Masson S, Fumagalli R, Pesenti A, Romero M, Fanizza C, Caspani L, Faenza S, Grasselli G, Iapichino G, Antonelli M, Parrini V, Fiore G, Latini R, Gattinoni L, ALBIOS Study Investigators: Albumin replacement in patients with severe sepsis or septic shock. N Engl J Med 2014; 370:1412–1421.

14 Perner A, Haase N, Guttormsen AB, Tenhunen J, Klemenzson G, Åneman A, Madsen KR, Møller MH, Elkjær JM, Poulsen LM, Bendtsen A, Winding R, Steensen M, Berezowicz P, Søe-Jensen P, Bestle M, Strand K, Wiis J, White JO, Thornberg KJ, Quist L, Nielsen J, Andersen LH, Holst LB, Thormar K, Kjældgaard AL, Fabritius ML, Mondrup F, Pott FC, Møller TP, Winkel P, Wetterslev J, 6S Trial Group, Scandinavian Critical Care Trials Group: Hydroxyethyl starch versus Ringer's acetate in severe sepsis. N Engl J Med 2012;367:124–134.

15 Myburgh JA, Finfer S, Bellomo R, Billot L, Cass A, Gattas D, Glass P, Lipman J, Liu B, McArthur C, McGuinness S, Rajbhandari D, Taylor CB, Webb SA, CHEST Investigators, Australian and New Zealand Intensive Care Society Clinical Trials Group: Hydroxyethyl starch or saline for fluid resuscitation in intensive care. N Engl J Med 2012;367:1901–1911.

16 Dickenmann M, Oettl T, Mihatsch MJ: Osmotic nephrosis: acute kidney injury with accumulation of proximal tubular lysosomes due to administration of exogenous solutes. Am J Kidney Dis 2008;51:491–503.

17 KDIGO AKI Work Group: KDIGO clinical practice guideline for acute kidney injury. Kidney Int Suppl 2012;2:1–138.

18 Wilcox CS: Regulation of renal blood flow by plasma chloride. J Clin Invest 1983;71:726–735.

19 Bullivant EM, Wilcox CS, Welch WJ: Intrarenal vasoconstriction during hyperchloremia: role of thromboxane. Am J Physiol 1989;256:F152–F157.

20 Chowdhury AH, Cox EF, Francis ST, Lobo DN: A randomized, controlled, double-blind crossover study on the effects of 2-L infusions of 0.9% saline and plasma-lyte® 148 on renal blood flow velocity and renal cortical tissue perfusion in healthy volunteers. Ann Surg 2012;256:18–24.

21 McCluskey SA, Karkouti K, Wijeysundera D, Minkovich L, Tait G, Beattie WS: Hyperchloremia after noncardiac surgery is independently associated with increased morbidity and mortality: a propensity-matched cohort study. Anesth Analg 2013;117:412–421.

22 Raghunathan K, Shaw A, Nathanson B, Stürmer T, Brookhart A, Stefan MS, Setoguchi S, Beadles C, Lindenauer PK: Association between the choice of IV crystalloid and in-hospital mortality among critically ill adults with sepsis. Crit Care Med 2014;42:1585–1591.

23 Yunos NM, Bellomo R, Hegarty C, Story D, Ho L, Bailey M: Association between a chloride-liberal vs chloride-restrictive intravenous fluid administration strategy and kidney injury in critically ill adults. JAMA 2012;308:1566–1572.

24 ProCESS Investigators, Yealy DM, Kellum JA, Huang DT, Barnato AE, Weissfeld LA, Pike F, Terndrup T, Wang HE, Hou PC, LoVecchio F, Filbin MR, Shapiro NI, Angus DC: A randomized trial of protocol-based care for early septic shock. The ProCESS investigators. N Engl J Med 2014;370:1683–1693.

25 ARISE Investigators, ANZICS Clinical Trials Group, Peake SL, Delaney A, Bailey M, Bellomo R, Cameron PA, Cooper DJ, Higgins AM, Holdgate A, Howe BD, Webb SA, Williams P: Goal-directed resuscitation for patients with early septic shock. N Engl J Med 2014;371:1496–1506.

26 Mouncey PR, Osborn TM, Power GS, Harrison DA, Sadique MZ, Grieve RD, Jahan R, Harvey SE, Bell D, Bion JF, Coats TJ, Singer M, Young JD, Rowan KM, ProMISe Trial Investigators: Trial of early, goal-directed resuscitation for septic shock. N Engl J Med 2015;372:1301–1311.

27 Asfar P, Meziani F, Hamel JF, Grelon F, Megarbane B, Anguel N, Mira JP, Dequin PF, Gergaud S, Weiss N, Legay F, Le Tulzo Y, Conrad M, Robert R, Gonzalez F, Guitton C, Tamion F, Tonnelier JM, Guezennec P, Van Der Linden T, Vieillard-Baron A, Mariotte E, Pradel G, Lesieur O, Ricard JD, Hervé F, du Cheyron D, Guerin C, Mercat A, Teboul JL, Radermacher P, SEPSISPAM Investigators: High versus low blood pressure target in patients with septic shock. N Engl J Med 2014;370:1583–1593.

28 Osman D, Ridel C, Ray P, Monnet X, Anguel N, Richard C, Teboul JL: Cardiac filling pressures are not appropriate to predict hemodynamic response to volume challenge. Crit Care Med 2007;35:64–68.

29 Michard F, Teboul JL: Predicting fluid responsiveness in ICU patients: a critical analysis of the evidence. Chest 2002;121:2000–2008.

30 Michard F, Boussat S, Chemla D, Anguel N, Mercat A, Lecarpentier Y, Richard C, Pinsky MR, Teboul JL: Relation between respiratory changes in arterial pulse pressure and fluid responsiveness in septic patients with acute circulatory failure. Am J Respir Crit Care Med 2000;162:134–138.

31 Michard F: Changes in arterial pressure during mechanical ventilation. Anesthesiology 2005;103:419–428.

32 Monnet X, Osman D, Ridel C, Lamia B, Richard C, Teboul JL: Predicting volume responsiveness by using the end-expiratory occlusion in mechanically ventilated intensive care unit patients. Crit Care Med 2009;37:951–956.
33 Monnet X, Rienzo M, Osman D, Anguel N, Richard C, Pinsky MR, Teboul JL: Passive leg raising predicts fluid responsiveness in the critically ill. Crit Care Med 2006;34:1402–1407.
34 Feissel M, Michard F, Faller JP, Teboul JL: The respiratory variation in inferior vena cava diameter as a guide to fluid therapy. Intensive Care Med 2004;30:1834–1837.
35 Vieillard-Baron A, Chergui K, Rabiller A, Peyrouset O, Page B, Beauchet A, Jardin F: Superior vena caval collapsibility as a gauge of volume status in ventilated septic patients. Intensive Care Med 2004;30:1734–1739.

Chiao-Lin Chuang, MD, PhD
Division of General Medicine, Department of Medicine
Taipei Veterans General Hospital
No. 201, Sec. 2, Shih-Pai Road, Taipei 112 (Taiwan)
E-Mail clchuang@vghtpe.gov.tw

AKI Management

# Multidimensional Approach to Adequacy of Renal Replacement Therapy in Acute Kidney Injury

Gianluca Villa[a] · Zaccaria Ricci[b] · Stefano Romagnoli[a–c] · Claudio Ronco[d]

[a]Department of Health Science, Section of Anaesthesiology and Intensive Care, University of Florence, Florence, [b]Department of Cardiology and Cardiac Surgery, Pediatric Cardiac Intensive Care Unit, Bambino Gesù Children's Hospital, IRCCS, Rome, [c]Department of Anaesthesia and Intensive Care, Azienda Ospedaliero-Universitaria Careggi, Florence, and [d]Department of Nephrology, Dialysis and Transplantation, and International Renal Research Institute, San Bortolo Hospital, Vicenza, Italy

## Abstract

Acute kidney injury (AKI) is frequently observed among hospitalized and critical care patients. In the absence of any effective therapies aiming to actively restore kidney function, AKI is usually managed through acute renal replacement therapy (ARRT). 'Optimization' of ARRT may reduce the mortality of patients with AKI. Although several studies have tried to identify the most adequate approach to ARRT in terms of dose, treatment modality and all other important dimensions, the literature has provided controversial results. Nowadays, adequate ARRT still appears difficult to dose, prescribe, deliver and monitor among different critical care patients. The identification of the major elements involved for a multidimensional approach to adequacy of ARRT in patients with AKI should consider the patient, the applied technology and the environment. All these aspects should be carefully evaluated and adequately applied in clinical practice through a patient-oriented approach. Adequacy of ARRT imposes the concomitant consideration of more complex issues, such as the timing, modality and technique of ARRT delivery; anticoagulation and substitution fluid choice; membrane selection; monitor accuracy; the role of fluid overload; and other patient comorbidities. The capacity of clinicians to consider all these aspects through a multidimensional approach, adapting the different dimensions of ARRT to actual patients' needs, might be the fundamental missing element in the pathway toward significant outcome improvements among critically ill patients with AKI. This narrative review provides a systematic approach to the major dimensions of ARRT and their multidimensional rationalization for adequate treatment prescription, monitoring and evaluation.

© 2016 S. Karger AG, Basel

## Introduction

Acute kidney injury (AKI) is a clinical syndrome characterized by an acute decrease in renal function, leading to retention of fluids and waste products [1]. It is frequently observed among hospitalized patients and intensive care unit (ICU) patients, with reported incidences of 5–7% and 25%, respectively [1, 2]. Evidence in the published literature shows that AKI is an independent risk factor for mortality, especially among critical care patients with multiorgan dysfunction [2]. Despite increasing knowledge about AKI physiopathology, the mortality rate related to this syndrome has not changed over time.

In the absence of any effective therapy aiming to actively restore kidney function, AKI is usually initially managed through conservative supportive treatments, such as optimization of fluid balance, correction of electrolyte and acid-base disturbances, dose adjustment of medications that are excreted by the kidneys, and prevention of secondary hemodynamic and nephrotoxic renal injuries [3]. However, approximately 6% of patients with AKI are treated with acute renal replacement therapy (ARRT) [2], which, beyond the conservative therapies, is essentially the only effective method for the management of critically ill patients with severe AKI [1, 2]. Within ARRT, several techniques of blood purification have been described for the management of critically ill patients, and among these, continuous ARRT (CRRT) is generally preferred for its distinctive hemodynamic tolerance and its efficacious removal of solutes and water [4–6].

It is currently recognized that 'optimization' of ARRT may reduce the mortality of patients with AKI [7]; in particular, an accurate evaluation of the timing, modality and dose of treatment might improve renal and nonrenal outcomes in these patients. The concept of adequacy during ARRT has been extensively reviewed in the last few years, and the literature suggests that an adequate treatment is one that closely reproduces the clearance of the kidneys [8].

## Multidimensional Approach to Adequacy of Acute Renal Replacement Therapy

Several studies have tried to identify the most adequate approach to ARRT, but ARRT still appears difficult to prescribe, deliver and monitor in critical care patients. In fact, for ARRT, there is no clinical consensus on the posology, treatment duration, or administration route with regard to a continuous or intermittent modality.

Adequacy of ARRT requires simultaneous consideration of several complex aspects, such as the timing, modality, and technique of ARRT delivery; the choice of anticoagulants and substitution fluids; membrane selection; and patient co-morbidities. The clinician's ability to consider these multiple aspects through a multidimensional approach might be the missing link between the provision of therapy and significant outcome improvements in critically ill AKI patients.

The major factors to be taken into consideration for a comprehensive approach to the management of AKI patients treated with ARRT are the patient, the applied technology and the environment.

In critical care patients, AKI is defined through clinical and biochemical parameters that assess renal function irrespective of the etiology. However, renal damage is usually a clinical manifestation of significant systemic damage. In fact, being the cause or consequence of one or more physiopathologic mechanisms (e.g. cardiorenal syndromes), AKI is generally inserted in a clinical picture of multiorgan dysfunction with a wide spectrum of clinical variability (e.g. sepsis). Therefore, to maximize the global patient outcome, it is of crucial importance to consider the direct and indirect consequences of ARRT on other organs while supporting renal function. Essential in this context is the multiparametric evaluation of patients with AKI throughout their ICU stay; for instance, the choice of continuous or intermittent ARRT may be based on systemic evaluation results, such as the presence of hemodynamic instability or physiotherapy requirements. Similar considerations should be made for all other dimensions of ARRT, as systemic conditions may lead to a need for a change in all other ARRT parameters, irrespective of renal-specific requirements.

The application of modern technology guarantees safe and feasible treatment, irrespective of the use of standard machines for intermittent hemodialysis (IHD) or of fourth-generation machines for CRRT. The high flexibility of these machines allows one to easily move from a pure dialytic technique (e.g. continuous veno-venous hemodialysis) to a pure convective technique (e.g. continuous veno-venous hemofiltration (CVVH)), passing through a range of mutually overlapping techniques (e.g. continuous veno-venous hemodiafiltration) according to patient requirements. The use of biofeedback, such as that for urea or blood volume variations during ARRT, allows for automatic modulation of the treatment parameters to adjust the clearance properties to the patient's physiologic variation observed during the extracorporeal therapy. Similarly, engineering improvements in machine hardware and software allow for automated or assisted guidance of treatment, such as in downtime dose compensation or calcium replacement during citrate anticoagulation. Nevertheless, all these technological applications should be carefully evaluated by the physician according to a physiopathologically oriented approach in order to individualize patient treatment.

Finally, the environment in which AKI patients undergo ARRT highly influences the feasibility and outcomes of treatment and should be considered for

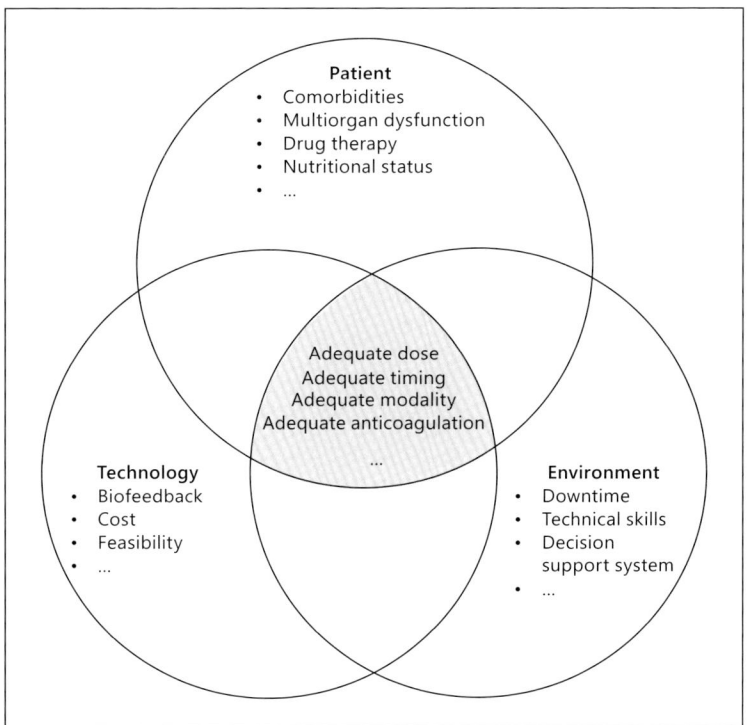

**Fig. 1.** The major factors to be taken into consideration for a comprehensive approach in the management of AKI patients treated with an ARRT.

adequate prescription, delivery and monitoring of this therapy. In particular, the technical and nontechnical skills of the staff involved in the management of ARRT as well as the downtime related to the center and the patient needs (e.g. radiological evaluation) should all be considered in treatment phases.

Although it is essential to take these 3 factors into consideration for a multidimensional approach, the bed-side practical application of ARRT requires the break-down of the whole treatment into its individual parameters for a pragmatic and systematic approach (see fig. 1).

## Dose

Set in the prescription phase and continuously monitored during treatment, the dialytic dose represents the 'posology' of ARRT; it usually identifies the efficiency (or clearance) of the treatment, which is defined as the amount of blood cleared by the renal replacement therapy over a given period of time [9]. This specific concept should be applied to a particular solute, and it does not represent actual mass removal, but rather its value normalized to the solute serum concentration. The intensity of treatment represents the clearance obtained during the effective time of treatment [9]. It is usually affected by the observed downtime, which significantly decreases the effective time of treatment and leads to a significant difference between the prescribed and the actually delivered doses. Finally, the efficacy of the treatment represents the ratio between the intensity and the volume of distribution of the marker solute [9]. In patients with chronic kidney disease treated with hemodialysis, all these variables might be directly measured and correlate with long-term outcomes [10]. In contrast, in patients with AKI treated with ARRT in the ICU, these variables are usually estimated through the flows set in the ARRT machine [11]. The errors obtained with this easy-to-use and feasible simplification should be taken into account to adapt the treatment performance to the specific patient. In particular, the amount of predilution used affects the linear relationship between clearance and the effluent rate; the downtime is not usually considered within this dose estimation; and finally, the progressive physiologic performance reduction of the membrane (i.e. membrane fouling) affects the solutes cleared by the effluent. Furthermore, although in patients with chronic kidney disease, urea is the marker solute used to quantify the efficacy of treatment, other large solutes may be more appropriate for ICU patients, such as inflammatory mediators or myoglobin.

Several studies observed a direct correlation between dose and the outcome of critical care patients [12]. However, although higher doses are considered the most adequate for these patients [12], recent large studies have disproved this concept. Indeed, the RENAL [13] and the ATN [14] studies have not observed any differences in terms of outcome between patients treated with a 'more intensive dose' (40 and 35 ml/kg/h, respectively) and patients treated with a 'less intensive dose' (25 and 20 ml/kg/h, respectively) [15]. Similar results have been observed when comparing large multicenter databases of AKI patients treated with different doses [16].

Nowadays, the most adequate dose is clinically recognized to be one that, if further increased, does not produce a direct improvement in patient outcome [3, 8]. However, it is important to consider that if low doses are used, this may lead to undertreatment and worse outcomes, whereas high doses may increase the clearance of nutrients and antibiotics, the cost of the treatment [17] and the risk of electrolyte disorders.

Considering all these points, the identification of an adequate dose range is critically important. Although the most recent clinical guidelines on AKI recommend delivering an effluent volume of 20–25 ml/kg/h for CRRT in AKI [18], nowadays, an actual delivery dose between 20 and 35 ml/kg/h is considered

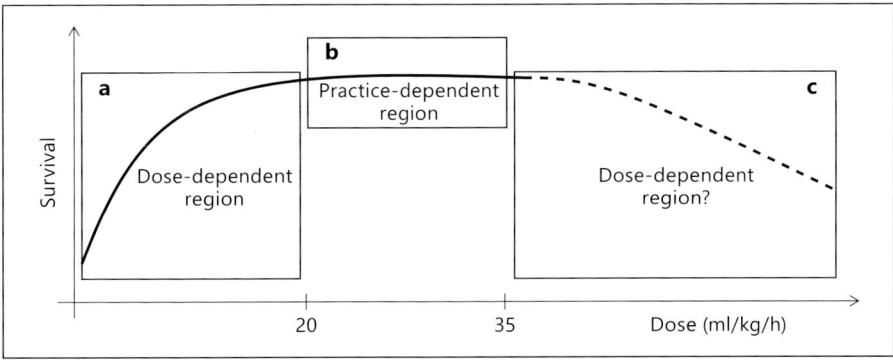

**Fig. 2.** Correlation between dose and outcome. When increasing the dose up to 20 ml/kg/h (**a**), the higher the dose obtained during renal replacement therapy, the higher the patient survival observed (dose-dependent region). A further increase in the dose prescription up to 35 ml/kg/h (**b**) may not influence the patient's survival. In contrast, other variables, such as the time of treatment and the optimization of blood perfusion or drug adjustments, may influence the outcome (practice-dependent region). When the prescribed dose is further increased (over 35 ml/kg/h, (**c**)), the patient may be prone to electrolyte disorders and to removal of nutrients and drugs (e.g. antibiotics), potentially reducing survival.

clinically acceptable [16]. In particular, within this dose range, patient survival does not depend on the specific delivered dose, but rather mainly on other variables, such as timing, patient characteristics, comorbidities or concomitant supportive pharmacologic therapies (practice-dependent region). In contrast, under 20 ml/kg/h and over 35 ml/kg/h, the outcome is dose dependent, and a direct correlation between dose and survival is observed [3, 8] (see fig. 2).

## Timing of Initiation

Numerous attempts have been made to define the most appropriate timing for ARRT initiation, particularly among critically ill patients with AKI [19]. However, adequate timing of ARRT initiation has not been exactly identified so far [3]; the current decision to initiate ARRT is still based on clinical or biochemical features of fluid overload and/or accumulation of waste solutes [18].

Most reasonably, beyond the 'rescue therapy' of renal substitution, proactive initiation of ARRT should be performed, mainly among critically ill patients with AKI. In particular, the preemptive initiation of ARRT might support (instead of completely replacing) kidney function during the early phases of organ dysfunction. ARRT might thus be modulated according to the pharmacologic treatment requirements and the different phases of metabolic and/or inflammatory clinical features of the patient observed during the ICU stay, reducing the further development of advanced complications.

However, only retrospective and observational cohort studies and small underpowered prospective trials [20] have suggested that an 'early' onset of renal replacement therapy might be associated with an improved outcome in patients with AKI [3]. Furthermore, the literature has failed to define what exactly 'early' is. In the first study suggesting a direct relationship between early onset and patient survival as well as in an observational study performed by the Program to Improve Care in Acute Renal Disease (PICARD) [21], the levels of blood urea or blood urea nitrogen were used to categorize the time of treatment [22]. Use of the timing between ARRT initiation and ICU admission has also been advocated to define the 'early' onset of extracorporeal treatment [23]. However, the staging of AKI at ARRT initiation, evaluated through clinical classifications, might be the most useful tool to identify 'early' and 'late' treatments [24].

Although conflicting results are available in the literature [20], in all these studies, an 'early' initiation of ARRT was significantly associated with an improvement in patient outcome. Furthermore, recent meta-analysis, including studies that comprehensively compared early and late onset of ARRT (independently of the used definition), suggested a positive effect for early initiation of extracorporeal treatment on patient survival [25, 26].

**Treatments and Modalities**

The modality applied during ARRT does not seem to affect the mortality rate of patients with AKI [8]. However, the preference for intermittent or continuous application of the extracorporeal treatment is still highly debated in the literature, and the initial setting for ARRT is currently chosen according to treatment availability in the center, the technical skills of the operators and the patient's hemodynamic status [3]. Several studies suggest similar hospital mortality rates as well as similar ICU and hospital lengths of stay between patients treated with CRRT and patients treated with IHD [8]. However, the use of IHD as an initial treatment for ARRT has been demonstrated to be related to a lower rate of renal recovery and a high incidence of dialysis-dependent conditions [27, 28]. In particular, solute and fluid control is achieved within a few hours during IHD, with a subsequent rapid change in the patient's volemia and fluid and/or solute components among different body compartments [3]. In these cases, systemic hypotension occurs in approximately 20–30% of cases of IHD treatment [29], leading to reduction of renal blood flow and further worsening the kidney damage [8].

**Table 1.** Advantages and disadvantages for continuous and intermittent ARRT

|  | Intermittent ARRT | Continuous ARRT |
|---|---|---|
| Advantages | – Rapid removal of toxins and circulating solutes<br>– Reduced downtime for diagnostic and therapeutic procedures<br>– Reduced exposure to anticoagulation<br>– Lower cost than CRRT | – Continuous removal of toxins and solutes (avoids concentration rebound)<br>– Hemodynamic tolerability<br>– Easy control of fluid balance<br>– Avoidance of disequilibrium syndrome<br>– User-friendly machines |
| Disadvantages | – Rapid fluid removal and frequent hypotension<br>– Dialysis disequilibrium and risk of cerebral edema<br>– Technically complex | – Slower solute clearance than for IHD<br>– Need for prolonged anticoagulation<br>– Reduced patient mobilization<br>– Hypothermia<br>– Increased cost relative to IHD |

Compared to IHD, the lower solute clearance and the slower removal of fluid per unit of time achieved with CRRT allow CRRT better hemodynamic tolerance [1], particularly among critically ill patients. As a consequence, CRRT is currently suggested for patients with hemodynamic instability or those in whom large fluctuations of solute concentrations and fluid shifts should be avoided, such as during brain injury, endocranic hypertension or generalized brain edema [18] (see table 1).

Current evidence does not allow recommendation of a specific extracorporeal modality over another [3]. Theoretically, the diffusive clearance achieved during continuous veno-venous hemodialysis is negatively affected by the solute's molecular weight. In contrast, the convective clearance achieved during CVVH is mainly affected by intrinsic properties of the membrane, such as the ultrafiltration coefficient. Because extracorporeal removal of small solutes, such as urea and creatinine, is of limited interest during early renal support therapy in the ICU, many clinicians prefer to use CVVH for critically ill patients with AKI. In this context, convective clearance may effectively attenuate the systemic inflammatory response syndrome by removing middle-molecular-weight molecules, such as cytokines.

## Anticoagulation

An appropriate anticoagulation approach is critically important during ARRT and is tightly related to treatment delivery and to the individualization of the prescription during ARRT. In particular, data from the literature have shown a

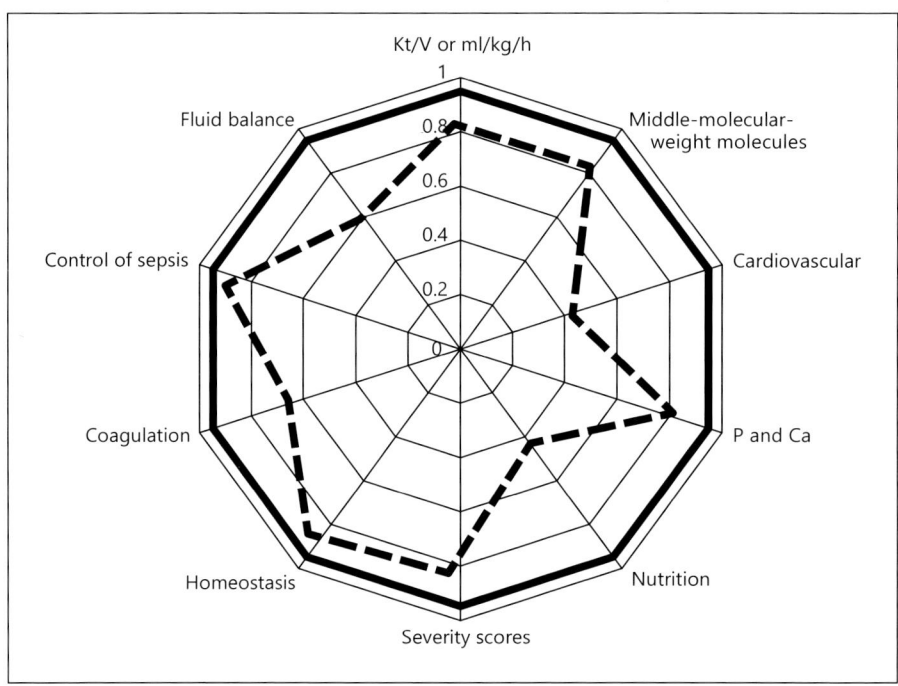

**Fig. 3.** Different parameters are considered to define a treatment as adequate. Maximal effort should be made to achieve a rounded shape in the final graph, in which every parameter is optimized (solid line, nearly adequate; dotted line, clearly inadequate).

relationship between the anticoagulation strategy and the efficacy of solute clearance and/or circuit longevity [30]. Although systemic anticoagulation and regional anticoagulation are both potentially efficacious in reducing membrane fouling due to the filter clotting, the use of regional citrate seems to be significantly associated with a prolonged filter life and with increased efficacy in term of the delivered dose compared to heparin or no anticoagulation [30].

Although membrane fouling affects the transmembrane clearance via a predictable mechanism involving filter clotting and clogging, it is not easily quantifiable in clinical practice. The clearance of urea is usually utilized to quantify the clearance properties of the treatment. Unfortunately, urea is a 60-Dalton non-protein-bound molecule that unreliably describes the kinetics of other molecules, especially in the ICU, where the target solutes are often middle-molecular-weight molecules, such as inflammatory mediators. In this context, an accurate anticoagulation strategy should be performed to ensure adequate transmembrane clearance of large molecules for a long period of time.

Although the Kidney Disease: Improving Global Outcomes guidelines identify regional citrate anticoagulation as the gold standard for anticoagulation in all patients without contraindication, independently of the risk of bleeding, the use of systemic unfractionated heparin remains the most common anticoagulation strategy during ARRT.

Among patients with an absolute contraindication to citrate administration, unfractionated or low-molecular-weight heparin has been identified as the most appropriate anticoagulation strategy in patients with a low risk of bleeding, while no anticoagulation is recommended for patients with a high risk of bleeding.

Finally, the use of other anticoagulants is currently recommended only for patients with heparin-induced thrombocytopenia; in these patients, direct thrombin inhibitors (such as argatroban) or Factor Xa inhibitors (such as danaparoid or fondaparinux) should be preferred over no anticoagulation strategy during ARRT [18].

## Conclusions

The management of patients with AKI may be particularly complex and requires a multidisciplinary and multiparametric approach. The delivery of adequate ARRT requires multidimensional consideration of the constantly changing clinical characteristics of the patient, the highly complex technology applied and the environment in which the treatment is administered. As a result, the physician should modulate the application of all ARRT dimensions in order to provide patient-individualized treatment. To better describe the concept, the radar graph shown in figure 3 can be utilized to evaluate the overall adequacy of a renal replacement therapy in the acute setting. To define a treatment as adequate, the graph should display a rounded shape, in which every parameter is optimized, as much as possible.

## References

1 Tolwani A: Continuous renal-replacement therapy for acute kidney injury. N Engl J Med 2012;367:2505–2514.
2 Uchino S, Kellum J, Bellomo R, Doig G, Morimatsu H, Morgera S, et al: Acute renal failure in critically ill patients: a multinational, multicenter study. JAMA 2005;294:813–818.
3 Villa G, Ricci Z, Ronco C: Renal replacement therapy. Crit Care Clin 2015;31:839–848.
4 Davenport A, Will E, Davidson A: Improved cardiovascular stability during continuous modes of renal replacement therapy in critically ill patients with acute hepatic and renal failure. Crit Care Med 1993;21:328–338.
5 Uchino S, Bellomo R, Ronco C: Intermittent versus continuous renal replacement therapy in the ICU: impact on electrolyte and acid-base balance. Intensive Care Med 2001;27:1037–1043.

6 Swartz RD, Messana JM, Orzol S, Port FK: Comparing continuous hemofiltration with hemodialysis in patients with severe acute renal failure. Am J Kidney Dis 1999;34:424–432.

7 Kellum JA, Mehta RL, Levin A, Molitoris BA, Warnock DG, Shah SV, et al: Development of a clinical research agenda for acute kidney injury using an international, interdisciplinary, three-step modified delphi process. Clin J Am Soc Nephrol 2008;3:887–894.

8 Ricci Z, Romagnoli S, Villa G, Ronco C: Modality and dosing of acute renal replacement therapy. Minerva Urol Nefrol 2015, Epub ahead of print.

9 Ricci Z, Bellomo R, Ronco C: Dose of dialysis in acute renal failure. Clin J Am Soc Nephrol 2006;1:380–388.

10 Ronco C, Brendolan A, Crepaldi C, Dissegna D, Gastaldon F, Ghezzi PM, et al: Measurement of effective delivery of the prescribed dialysis treatment. Nephrol Dial Transpl 1996;11:68–74.

11 Uchino S, Bellomo R, Morimatsu H, Morgera S, Schetz M, Tan I, et al: Continuous renal replacement therapy: a worldwide practice survey. The beginning and ending supportive therapy for the kidney (B.E.S.T. kidney) investigators. Intensive Care Med 2007;33:1563–1570.

12 Ronco C, Bellomo R, Homel P, Brendolan A, Dan M, Piccinni P, et al: Effects of different doses in continuous veno-venous haemofiltration on outcomes of acute renal failure: a prospective randomised trial. Lancet 2000;356:26–30.

13 RENAL Replacement Therapy Study Investigators; Bellomo R, Cass A, Cole L, Finfer S, Gallagher M, et al: Intensity of continuous renal-replacement therapy in critically ill patients. N Engl J Med 2009;361:1627–1638.

14 VA/NIH Acute Renal Failure Trial Network; Palevsky P, Zhang J, O'Connor T, Chertow G, Crowley S, et al: Intensity of renal support in critically ill patients with acute kidney injury. N Engl J Med 2008;359:7–20.

15 Ricci Z, Ronco C: Timing, dose and mode of dialysis in acute kidney injury. Curr Opin Crit Care 2011;17:556–561.

16 Uchino S, Toki N, Takeda K, Ohnuma T, Namba Y, Katayama S, et al: Validity of low-intensity continuous renal replacement therapy. Crit Care Med 2013;41:2584–2591.

17 Rimmelé T, Kellum JA: Clinical review: blood purification for sepsis. Crit Care 2011;15:205.

18 Kidney Disease: Improving Global Outcomes (KDIGO) Acute Kidney Injury Work Group: KDIGO clinical practice guideline for acute kidney injury. Kidney Int Suppl 2012;2:1–138.

19 Zaragoza JJ, Villa G, Garzotto F, Sharma A, Lorenzin A, Ribeiro L, et al: Initiation of renal replacement therapy in the intensive care unit in Vicenza (IRRIV) score. Blood Purif 2015;39:246–257.

20 Bouman CS, Oudemans-Van Straaten HM, Tijssen JG, Zandstra DF, Kesecioglu J: Effects of early high-volume continuous venovenous hemofiltration on survival and recovery of renal function in intensive care patients with acute renal failure: a prospective, randomized trial. Crit Care Med 2002;30:2205–2211.

21 Liu KD, Himmelfarb J, Paganini E, Ikizler TA, Soroko SH, Mehta RL, et al: Timing of initiation of dialysis in critically ill patients with acute kidney injury. Clin J Am Soc Nephrol 2006;1:915–919.

22 Palevsky P: Renal replacement therapy in AKI. Adv Chronic Kidney Dis 2013;20:76–84.

23 Bagshaw SM, Uchino S, Bellomo R, Morimatsu H, Morgera S, Schetz M, et al: Timing of renal replacement therapy and clinical outcomes in critically ill patients with severe acute kidney injury. J Crit Care 2009;24:129–140.

24 Shiao C-C, Wu V-C, Li W-Y, Lin Y-F, Hu F-C, Young G-H, et al: Late initiation of renal replacement therapy is associated with worse outcomes in acute kidney injury after major abdominal surgery. Crit Care 2009;13:R171.

25 Karvellas CJ, Farhat MR, Sajjad I, Mogensen SS, Leung A, Wald R, et al: A comparison of early versus late initiation of renal replacement therapy in critically ill patients with acute kidney injury: a systematic review and meta-analysis. Crit Care 2011;15:R72.

26 Wang X, Yuan WJ: Timing of initiation of renal replacement therapy in acute kidney injury: a systematic review and meta-analysis. Ren Fail 2012;34:396–402.

27 Schneider AG, Bellomo R, Bagshaw SM, Glassford NJ, Lo S, Jun M, et al: Choice of renal replacement therapy modality and dialysis dependence after acute kidney injury: a systematic review and meta-analysis. Intensive Care Med 2013;39:987–997.

28 Wald R, Shariff SZ, Adhikari NKJ, Bagshaw SM, Burns KE, Friedrich JO, et al: The association between renal replacement therapy modality and long-term outcomes among critically ill adults with acute kidney injury: a retrospective cohort study. Crit Care Med 2013;42:1–10.

29 Selby NM, McIntyre CW: A systematic review of the clinical effects of reducing dialysate fluid temperature. Nephrol Dial Transplant 2006;21:1883–1898.

30 Claure-del Granado R, Macedo E, Soroko S, Kim Y, Chertow GM, Himmelfarb J, et al: Anticoagulation, delivered dose and outcomes in CRRT: the program to improve care in acute renal disease (PICARD). Hemodial Int 2014;18:641–649.

Claudio Ronco, MD, Director
Department of Nephrology Dialysis and Transplantation
International Renal Research Institute (IRRIV), San Bortolo Hospital
Viale Rodolfi, 37, IT–36100 Vicenza (Italy)
E-Mail cronco@goldnet.it

# Timing of Renal Replacement Therapy in Acute Kidney Injury

Marlies Ostermann[a] · Ron Wald[b] · Sean M. Bagshaw[c]

[a]Department of Critical Care and Nephrology, Guy's and St. Thomas Hospital, London, UK; [b]Division of Nephrology, St. Michael's Hospital, Toronto, Ont., and [c]Division of Critical Care Medicine, Faculty of Medicine and Dentistry, University of Alberta, Edmonton, Alta., Canada

## Abstract

**Background:** Renal replacement therapy (RRT) is commonly and increasingly utilized in critically ill patients with severe acute kidney injury (AKI). The issue of when to start RRT in a critically ill patient with AKI has long troubled clinicians. **Summary:** Currently, there is a paucity of high-quality evidence to guide clinician decision-making on the optimal time to start RRT. This lack of evidence has translated into wide variation in treatment patterns and practices. In patients developing life-threatening complications of AKI, the decision to start RRT is largely indisputable; however, in the absence of such complications, the optimal thresholds to start RRT that translates into improved outcomes for patients are unknown. Available evidence from observational studies and clinical trials have considerable limitations for translation to clinical practice due to their retrospective, post hoc secondary design, their small sample sizes, heterogeneity in study populations and illness severity, variation in the definitions of AKI and in the timing of or thresholds for starting RRT and the risk of residual confounding and bias related to the association between the timing of RRT and outcome. **Key Messages:** Several large randomized trials are planned or ongoing, and the results of these trials will greatly inform best clinical practice and will help reduce unnecessary variation in the practice of RRT prescription. For now, the decision on the appropriate time to start RRT is naturally complex, integrating numerous variables, and should largely be individualized.

© 2016 S. Karger AG, Basel

Acute kidney injury (AKI) is a common and increasingly encountered complication of critical illness that occurs in more than 50% of patients admitted to the intensive care unit (ICU) [1]. Among those with more severe AKI and those developing overt complications of AKI, renal replacement therapy (RRT) is often commenced [1, 2].

The issue of the appropriate time to start RRT in a critically ill patient with AKI has troubled clinicians for decades. The optimal threshold indicating when and in whom to commence RRT remains uncertain and is currently a high research priority in the field of critical care nephrology [3–5]. Among patients faced with life-threatening complications of AKI such as severe hyperkalemia, marked metabolic acidosis, and/or fluid overload, the decision to urgently start RRT is generally unequivocal (table 1). However, recent data have suggested that life-threatening complications attributable to AKI are less common reasons for critically ill AKI patients to receive RRT [6]. Indeed, in the absence of overt or impending life-threatening complications, the optimal time to start RRT is unknown [4, 5, 7, 8]. Not surprisingly, given this knowledge gap, there remains wide variation in clinical practice for the prescription of acute RRT in critical care settings [8–10]. Unfortunately, this variation likely contributes to inconsistent and suboptimal quality of care.

RRT does not truly replace kidney function; rather, RRT provides homeostatic support, often in the context of multi-organ injury and failure, as well as time to allow renal recovery to occur [11]. Accordingly, the goals of RRT are to achieve and maintain fluid, electrolyte, acid-base, and uremic solute homeostasis and to facilitate additional supportive measures when indicated (i.e., nutritional support, obligatory fluid intake, blood transfusions) while preventing the occurrence of overt life-threatening complications of AKI. Importantly, given the delicate nature of kidney-organ interactions (i.e., kidney-lung, kidney-heart, kidney-brain interactions) in critically ill states, RRT also provides an additional important form of multi-organ support by limiting the worsening of nonrenal organ dysfunction, which may be exacerbated by AKI and overt kidney failure [12].

## Impact of Renal Replacement Therapy on Outcomes

RRT, along with mechanical ventilation and vasoactive therapy, represent core life-sustaining technologies for critically ill patients. An estimated 8–10% of critically ill patients receive RRT, and this percentage is smaller than the percentage of critically ill patients who receive mechanical ventilation or vasoactive support. However, recent data have shown that the utilization of RRT has increased significantly [13]. Importantly, the initiation of RRT clearly represents an escalation in both the complexity and the cost of care. Patients with severe AKI receiving RRT are at increased risk for major morbidities, including nonrecovery of

**Table 1.** Summary of absolute and relative indications and contraindications for starting RRT in critically ill patients with AKI

| Absolute indications (in the absence of contraindications to RRT) | – Refractory hyperkalemia ($K^+$ >6.5 mmol/l, rapidly rising, or associated with cardiac toxicity)<br>– Refractory metabolic acidosis (pH ≤7.2 despite normal or low arterial $pCO_2$)<br>– Refractory pulmonary edema due to fluid overload unresponsive to diuretic therapy<br>– Symptoms or complications attributable to uremia (e.g., bleeding, pericarditis, or encephalopathy)<br>– Overdose/toxicity from a dialyzable drug/toxin |
|---|---|
| Relative indications (in the absence of life-threatening complications of AKI) | – Limited physiological reserve to tolerate the consequences of AKI<br>– Advanced nonrenal organ dysfunction exacerbated by excessive fluid accumulation (e.g., impaired respiratory function)<br>– Anticipated solute burden (e.g., tumor lysis syndrome; rhabdomyolysis; intravascular hemolysis)<br>– Need for administration of a large volume of fluid (e.g., nutritional support, medications or blood products)<br>– Severity of the underlying disease<br>– Concomitant accumulation of poisons or toxic drugs that can be removed by RRT (e.g., salicylates, ethylene glycol, methanol, metformin) |
| Relative contraindications | – Futile prognosis<br>– Patient receiving palliative care<br>– High likelihood of nonrecovery of renal function in a patient who is not a candidate for long-term dialysis |

AKI = Acute kidney injury; CKD = chronic kidney disease; RRT = renal replacement therapy.

kidney function, rapid progression to end-stage kidney disease and long-term dialysis dependence, and mortality [2, 14–16].

Circumstantial data have further suggested any receipt of RRT *per se* is independently associated with mortality among critically ill patients with AKI [9, 17]. While these observational data may suffer from a number of potential methodological limitations and biases, there is rationale for a potential association of RRT with increased risk for a poor outcome after adjustment for important confounders such as study cohort homogeneity and illness severity [18]. For example, the increased utilization of RRT among patients with a very low probability of survival due to a high burden of pre-morbid diseases and/or high illness severity may represent an important source of bias when evaluating the association of RRT with outcome [19]. Similarly, patients with less severe AKI who initially receive RRT for iatrogenic complications (i.e., unnecessary or excessive potassium supplementation) or marginal indications in which recovery was likely may also bias the association of RRT with outcome [20]. More recent data from observational studies in critically ill patients who develop conventional complications of AKI have shown a survival benefit from RRT initiation [21, 22].

**Table 2.** Benefits and drawbacks of early RRT in critically ill patients with AKI

| Benefits | Drawbacks |
| --- | --- |
| 'Unloading' or 'resting' stressed and damaged kidneys | Need for and complications associated with dialysis catheter insertion (e.g., bleeding, pneumothorax, and bloodstream infection) |
| Avoidance and/or earlier control of complications of uremia | Need for and complications associated with anticoagulation regimens |
| Avoidance and/or earlier control of electrolyte/metabolic derangement | Risk of iatrogenic episodes of hemodynamic instability that may exacerbate AKI and impede kidney repair/recovery |
| Avoidance and/or earlier control of acid-base imbalance | Risk of excess loss of unmeasured micronutrients and trace elements |
| Avoidance and/or early control of fluid accumulation and overload | Risk of excess clearance of vital medications (e.g., antimicrobials and anti-epileptics) below therapeutic levels |
| Avoidance of unnecessary diuretic exposure | Unnecessary exposure of patients who will spontaneously recover kidney function with conservative management to RRT |
| Immunomodulation and clearance of inflammatory mediators | Increased bedside workload for providers |
|  | Increased resource use and direct health costs |

AKI = Acute kidney injury; RRT = renal replacement therapy.

This may go so far as to limit the kidney's exposure to nephrotoxins or unnecessary high-dose diuretic therapy [33]. The ability of RRT to modulate inflammation/immune function in septic states is theoretically attractive but remains controversial [34]. The practice of starting RRT earlier in critically ill patients with AKI would appear, at face value, to confer a variety of benefits and is supported by circumstantial data and selected clinical trials [23, 24, 35–37].

Alternatively, there are potential concerns about starting RRT too early in the absence of clear indications (table 2). Patients receiving RRT will require central venous catheter insertion, blood exposure to an extracorporeal circuit, and anticoagulation regimens, each of which is recognized to be associated with adverse events. Importantly, exposure to iatrogenic episodes of hemodynamic instability may disrupt the kidney repair process and impede recovery [38]. Several studies have shown no clinical benefit from earlier initiation of RRT among patients with AKI [28, 39, 40]. Indeed, there is a paucity of high-quality evidence from RCTs confirming that starting RRT patients with AKI without life-threatening complications improves clinically important outcomes such as renal recovery or survival. Accordingly, the perceived benefits of starting RRT naturally

## Defining the Timing of Renal Replacement Therapy

There is no widely accepted or consensus-driven definition of the appropriate timing of RRT initiation for AKI. Studies to date have applied a broad range of definitions across a wide variety of study methodologies using terms such as 'early', 'accelerated', 'delayed', 'late' and 'standard' initiation of RRT [23–25]. It is important to acknowledge that the terms 'early' and 'late' are relative and that what may represent 'early' RRT in one clinical context for a given patient may in fact be 'late' for another patient with a distinct profile of clinical characteristics, diagnosis and illness severity. These definitions have integrated physiological parameters (e.g., urine output), biochemical parameters (e.g., serum creatinine and urea), timing relative to the development of AKI (which has also been variably defined), timing relative to hospital or ICU admission, and timing relative to the development of a complication of AKI or 'conventional' indications for starting RRT such as hyperkalemia, acidosis or fluid overload [6, 7, 22, 26–30]. This heterogeneity in how the timing of and the threshold for starting RRT, in particular what constitutes 'early', has presented significant challenges and has represented a fundamental barrier to progress in this field. Moreover, the majority of studies that have evaluated the timing of RRT in AKI patients have failed to consider patients with AKI who did not receive RRT [18]. It is plausible that a conservative strategy consisting of supportive management, watchful waiting, and initiation of RRT only when a life-threatening complication develops may indeed result in the spontaneous recovery of kidney function by patients with severe AKI. Indeed, this was recently shown in a Canadian multicenter pilot randomized controlled trial (RCT), in which 25% of patients randomized to a strategy of standard initiation of RRT recovered kidney function without receiving RRT [31].

## Rationale Concerning the Timing of Renal Replacement Therapy Initiation

There is rationale for a potential benefit of accelerated initiation of RRT among critically ill patients, particularly if the clinician's impression is that AKI is likely to worsen [32]. Earlier RRT may confer more rapid correction of electrolyte and acid-base derangements, better control or avoidance of complications of uremia, and mitigation of excessive fluid accumulation (table 2). Certainly, earlier RRT would prevent overt complications of AKI from occurring [21]. Theoretically, RRT may unload damaged and impaired kidneys providing it an opportunity to 'rest' and perhaps facilitating its recovery and repair. This would be analogous to providing mechanical ventilation to patients with acute lung injury.

be inappropriate due to a priori stated preferences for care from the patient or family or due the perception of a futile medical prognosis for a patient nearing end of life, in which RRT would not influence outcome. In these circumstances, withholding RRT would constitute good clinical practice and end-of-life care [42].

**Recent Clinical Studies of the Timing of Renal Replacement Therapy**

A number of studies of variable methodological quality and rigor have evaluated the thresholds for the timing of RRT in AKI patients. A summary of randomized trials is shown in table 3. Evidence syntheses of mostly observational studies have suggested that earlier RRT may improve survival [23, 24, 37]. However, inferences from the available observational data are limited because the study design was retrospective or post hoc, the study cohort was heterogeneous, the definitions of AKI and the thresholds or timing of RRT were distinct and the association between RRT timing and outcome displayed a relatively high risk of bias. As mentioned before, most observational studies did not compare AKI patients receiving RRT with AKI patients who did not receive RRT. One exception is a recent secondary analysis of the Finnish AKI (FINNAKI) study [22]. That study evaluated 239 critically ill patients treated with RRT and focused on the timing of RRT relative to development of one or more 'conventional' indications, including hyperkalemia, severe acidemia, uremia, oligoanuria and fluid overload with pulmonary edema. Timing was classified as 'pre-emptive' if RRT was started in the absence of these criteria; 'classic – urgent' if started within 12 h of developing one of these indications; and 'classic – delayed' if started more than 12 h after developing one of these indications. Based on multivariate and propensity-adjusted analyses, pre-emptive RRT was associated with lower 90-day mortality than RRT after the development of a classic indication (30 vs. 49%; odds ratio 2.1; 95% CI, 1.0–4.1). In addition, 90-day mortality was lower among patients treated with 'classic – urgent' RRT than among those treated with 'classic – delayed' RRT (39 vs. 68%; odds ratio 3.9; 95% CI, 1.5–10.2). Moreover, the mortality rate of AKI patients receiving pre-emptive RRT was lower than that of AKI patients not receiving RRT based on propensity-adjusted analysis.

Of the few RCTs that have evaluated the timing of RRT, all are small, underpowered and lack generalizability to truly inform whether hastening or reducing the threshold for starting RRT impacts clinically important patient-centered outcomes (table 3). The largest RCT reported to date included 208 hospitalized patients with community-acquired AKI who were randomized to early RRT, defined as RRT initiation upon a serum urea level >23 mmol/l or a serum

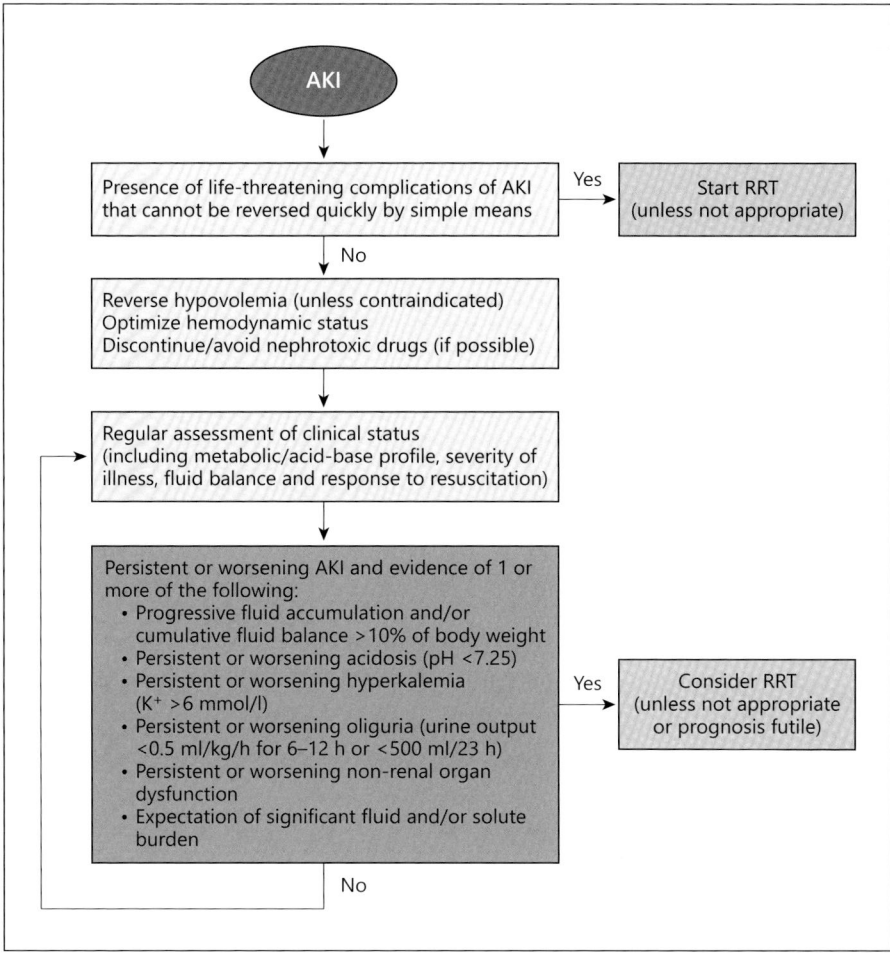

**Fig. 1.** Proposed algorithm to help decide when to initiate renal replacement therapy in critically ill patients with acute kidney injury.

have to be balanced with resource implications and the potential for harm within the context of the patient's and family's preferences for care [20, 41].

Figure 1 shows an algorithm that serves to aid clinicians in the decision-making process regarding when to consider starting RRT [25]. The main message is that the decision to start RRT should be individualized and based on the dynamic context and trajectory of the patient, integrating baseline clinical information (i.e., chronic kidney disease and renal reserve), acute diagnosis, illness severity, nonrenal organ dysfunction, and physiological and laboratory data rather than relying on absolute or arbitrary threshold values for laboratory tests [25]. Finally, it is important to consider that starting RRT in many patients may

**Table 3.** Summary of randomized controlled trials investigating the timing of RRT

| Study | Time period | Size | RRT modality | Patient population | Intervention early RRT | control treatment | Outcome (early RRT vs. control treatment) | Additional comments |
|---|---|---|---|---|---|---|---|---|
| Conger et al. [45] | Vietnam war (pre-1975) | n = 18 SC | IHD | Adult Major trauma | Urea >17.8 mmol/l or SCr >442 µmol/l | Urea >42.8 mmol/l or SCr >884 µmol/l | Mortality: 38 vs. 80% | – |
| Pursnani et al. [46] | N/A | n = 35 SC | IHD | Adult Medical/ obstetrical | Urea >42.8 mmol/l or SCr >619 µmol/l | Clinical decision | Mortality: 22 vs. 29% | ↓ Complications and length of hospital stay in the early RRT group |
| Sugahara et al. [36] | 1995–1997 | n = 28 SC | PIRRT | Adult Cardiac surgery | UO <30 ml/h × 3 h and SCr <44 µmol/l/ day | UO <20 ml/h × 2 h and SCr >44 µmol/l/ day | Mortality (14 days): 14 vs. 86% (p < 0.01) | 2 patients in the 'early' RRT group were still on RRT at day 14 |
| Durmaz et al. [35] | 1999–2001 | n = 44 SC | IHD | Adult CKD Cardiac surgery | 10% ↑ SCr from pre-operative value | ≥50% rise in SCr or UO <400 ml/24 h | Mortality: 5 vs. 30% (p = 0.048) | ↓ Complications and length of ICU stay in the early RRT group |
| Bouman et al. [39] | 1998–2000 | n = 106 2 centers | CVVH | Adult Critically ill Shock | UO <30 ml/h × 6 h and CrCl <20 ml/min | Urea >40 mmol/l or K$^+$ >6.5 mmol/l or pulmonary edema | Mortality (28 days): 29 vs. 25% (p = 0.8) Recovery: no difference | 4 patients in the control group recovered before RRT was started |

**Table 3.** Continued

| Study | Time period | Size | RRT modality | Patient population | Intervention early RRT | control treatment | Outcome (early RRT vs. control treatment) | Additional comments |
|---|---|---|---|---|---|---|---|---|
| Jamale et al. [40] | 2011–2012 | n = 208 SC | IHD | Adult Community-acquired AKI | Urea >25 mmol/l and/or SCr >619 μmol/l | Conventional indication for RRT (as per consensus decision by 2 nephrologists) | Mortality (hospital): 21 vs. 12% (p = 0.2) DD (3 months): 5 vs. 5% | In the control group, 13% recovered kidney function and 12% received emergency RRT |
| Wald et al. [31] | 2012–2014 | n = 100 MC | Mixed | Adult Critically ill | Two of SCr >2 × baseline; UO <6 ml/kg × 12 h; and blood NGAL >400 ng/ml | Conventional indication for RRT | Mortality (90 days): 38 vs. 37% DD (90 days): 0 vs. 6% | Trial design proven feasible |

AKI = Acute kidney injury; CKD = chronic kidney disease; RRT = renal replacement therapy; SC = single-center; MC = multi-center; CVVH = continuous venovenous hemofiltration; IHD = intermittent hemodialysis; PIRRT = prolonged intermittent renal replacement therapy; DD = dialysis dependence; UO = urine output; SCr = serum creatinine; NGAL = neutrophil gelatinase-associated lipocalin; UO = urine output; CrCl = creatinine clearance.

creatinine level >618 μmol/l, or standard care, defined as RRT initiation upon the detection of refractory hyperkalemia, acidosis or volume overload or in the setting of uremic symptoms [40]. No differences in mortality or recovery of kidney function were found between the groups. Recently, a pilot multi-center RCT, the Standard versus accelerated initiation of renal replacement therapy in AKI (STARRT-AKI) study, was completed [31]. This Canadian multi-center pilot RCT demonstrated the feasibility and safety of performing a definitive pragmatic approach of early/accelerated RRT compared to a conservative strategy (based on persistent AKI and/or the development of classic indications); however, this trial was not powered to inform on clinically important outcomes.

## Recommendations from Current Clinical Practice Guidelines

In 2012, the *Kidney Disease Improving Global Outcomes* (KDIGO) consortium and the *National Institute for Health and Care Excellence* (NICE) in the United Kingdom published official recommendations related to the timing of RRT initiation in patients with AKI [4, 5].

The KDIGO Clinical Practice Guideline (CPG) for AKI acknowledged that both the indications, in terms of clinical criteria and the patient-specific context, and the optimal time for starting RRT in patients with AKI were uncertain [4]. Accordingly, KDIGO provided the following consensus recommendations.

(i) Initiate RRT emergently when life-threatening changes in fluid, electrolyte, and acid-base balance exist (not rated).

(ii) Consider the broader clinical context, the presence of conditions that can be modified by RRT, and the trends of laboratory test results – rather than the blood urea nitrogen or creatinine threshold alone – when making the decision to start RRT (not rated).

The KDIGO CPG clearly recognizes that there is currently a paucity of high-quality evidence to provide strong recommendations for when to start RRT. Their statements further suggest that clinicians integrate not only the presence of life-threatening complications but also the broader clinical context of the patient, including the trajectory of illness severity, the burden of nonrenal organ dysfunction and the expectation concerning the likelihood that complications attributable to AKI will arise, into their decision-making on whether and when to start RRT.

Similarly, the NICE CPG for AKI [5] proposed the following recommendations regarding the timing of RRT initiation in patients with AKI; these recommendations were largely based on the findings from 2 RCTs and 3 prospective observational studies.

(i) Immediately discuss any potential indications for RRT with a nephrologist, a pediatric nephrologist and/or a critical care specialist to ensure that the therapy is started as soon as needed.

(ii) Immediately refer adults, children and young people for RRT if any of the following are not responding to medical management:
- Hyperkalemia
- Metabolic acidosis
- Complications of uremia (i.e., pericarditis, encephalopathy)
- Fluid overload
- Pulmonary edema.

(iii) Base the decision to start RRT on the condition of the adult, child or young person as a whole rather than on an isolated indicator such as the urea, creatinine or potassium level.

The NICE guidelines also acknowledge the paucity of high-quality evidence for guiding decision-making around this issue. The guidelines further emphasize that clinicians need better tools, such as clinical risk prediction scores or novel point of care tests (i.e., novel kidney damage biomarkers) that can incrementally discriminate patients who have a high likelihood of developing worsened AKI or a complication related to AKI and who may benefit from RRT from those who have a high likelihood of recovering kidney function and who may benefit from a conservative strategy because unnecessary RRT can be safely avoided.

**Future Randomized Clinical Trials**

There are currently four ongoing or planned randomized trials focused on generating high-quality evidence to guide the optimal timing of RRT initiation in critically ill patients with AKI. The Initiation of Dialysis EArly Versus Late in ICU (IDEAL-ICU) trial is a French multi-center RCT aiming to enroll 824 critically ill patients with septic shock and severe AKI (defined as a three-fold rise in the serum creatinine level and urine output <0.3 ml/kg/h for 12 h) [43]. That trial will compare a strategy of early RRT initiation, defined as RRT within 12 h of fulfilling AKI-based criteria, with a strategy of delayed RRT, defined as RRT 48–60 h after fulfilling AKI-based criteria. The Artificial Kidney Initiation in Kidney Injury (AKIKI) trial, another French multi-center RCT, proposes to enroll 620 critically ill patients with AKI randomized to either early RRT, defined as fulfilling the Failure category of the risk, injury, failure, loss, and end-stage kidney disease criteria, or a conservative strategy, defined as RRT initiation only after fulfilling the Failure category of the same criteria and an additional conventional indication for RRT [44]. The third trial is the Early versus late initiation of RRT in critically ill patients with AKI (ELAIN) trial, a recently completed (not yet reported) German multi-center RCT that enrolled 250 critically ill patients comparing the effect of early initiation of RRT, defined as RRT initiation upon fulfillment of the AKI Network classification of stage 2 AKI, and late RRT, defined as RRT initiation upon fulfillment of the AKI Network classification of stage 3 AKI or development of an absolute indication, on 90-day mortality (available at: file:///C:/data/Downloads/DRKS00004367_en%20(1).pdf) Finally, the STARRT-AKI trial will begin recruitment in late 2015. This is a Canadian-led multi-national RCT aiming to randomize 2,866 critically ill patients to accelerated RRT, defined as RRT initiation upon the predominant fulfillment of the KDIGO criteria for stage 2 AKI, or a conservative strategy, in which RRT is initiated for nonresolving AKI or following the development of complications, to compare the effects of these strategies on 90-day mortality.

These trials hold promise to greatly inform clinical practice.

## Conclusions

The evidence accumulated from observational studies and clinical trials to date has implied that the optimal time of RRT initiation in critically ill patients with AKI is uncertain. High-quality RCTs specifically focused on when to start RRT are ongoing, and the results will greatly inform best clinical practice. Such evidence is important for reducing unnecessary variations in the clinical practice of RRT prescription. For now, the decision on when to start RRT is naturally complex and should largely be individualized for a given patient-specific context whenever possible.

## References

1 Hoste EA, Bagshaw SM, Bellomo R, Cely CM, Colman R, Cruz DN, et al: Epidemiology of acute kidney injury in critically ill patients: the multinational AKI-EPI study. Intensive Care Med 2015;41:1411–1423.
2 Nisula S, Kaukonen KM, Vaara ST, Korhonen AM, Poukkanen M, Karlsson S, et al: Incidence, risk factors and 90-day mortality of patients with acute kidney injury in Finnish intensive care units: the FINNAKI study. Intensive Care Med 2013;39:420–428.
3 Joannidis M, Forni LG: Clinical review: timing of renal replacement therapy. Crit Care 2011;15:223.
4 Kidney Disease: Improving Global Outcomes (KDIGO) Acute Kidney Injury Work Group: KDIGO clinical practice guideline for acute kidney injury. Kidney International 2012; 2012(suppl):1–138.

5 National Institute for Health and Care Excellence Acute Kidney Injury Workgroup: Acute kidney injury: prevention, detection and management of acute kidney injury up to the point of renal replacement therapy. 2013. http://guidance.nice.org.uk/CG169/Guidance/pdf/English. (accessed December 20, 2014).

6 Bagshaw SM, Wald R, Barton J, Burns KE, Friedrich JO, House AA, et al: Clinical factors associated with initiation of renal replacement therapy in critically ill patients with acute kidney injury-a prospective multicenter observational study. J Crit Care 2012;27:268–275.

7 Bagshaw SM, Uchino S, Bellomo R, Morimatsu H, Morgera S, Schetz M, et al: Timing of renal replacement therapy and clinical outcomes in critically ill patients with severe acute kidney injury. J Crit Care 2009;24:129–140.

8 Clark E, Wald R, Levin A, Bouchard J, Adhikari NK, Hladunewich M, et al: Timing the initiation of renal replacement therapy for acute kidney injury in Canadian intensive care units: a multicentre observational study. Can J Anaesth 2012;59:861–870.

9 Elseviers MM, Lins RL, Van der Niepen P, Hoste E, Malbrain ML, Damas P, et al: Renal replacement therapy is an independent risk factor for mortality in critically ill patients with acute kidney injury. Crit Care 2010; 14:R221.

10 Ricci Z, Ronco C, D'Amico G, De Felice R, Rossi S, Bolgan I, et al: Practice patterns in the management of acute renal failure in the critically ill patient: an international survey. Nephrol Dial Transplant 2006;21:690–696.

11 Bagshaw SM, Wald R: Renal replacement therapy: when to start. Contrib Nephrol 2011; 174:232–241.

12 Bellomo R, Kellum JA, Ronco C: Acute kidney injury. Lancet 2012;380:756–766.

13 Wald R, McArthur E, Adhikari NK, Bagshaw SM, Burns KE, Garg AX, et al: Changing incidence and outcomes following dialysis-requiring acute kidney injury among critically ill adults: a population-based cohort study. Am J Kid Dis 2015;65:870–877.

14 Bagshaw SM, Laupland KB, Doig CJ, Mortis G, Fick GH, Mucenski M, et al: Prognosis for long-term survival and renal recovery in critically ill patients with severe acute renal failure: a population-based study. Crit Care 2005;9:R700–R709.

15 Uchino S, Kellum JA, Bellomo R, Doig GS, Morimatsu H, Morgera S, et al: Acute renal failure in critically ill patients: a multinational, multicenter study. JAMA 2005;294:813–818.

16 Wald R, Quinn RR, Luo J, Li P, Scales DC, Mamdani MM, et al: Chronic dialysis and death among survivors of acute kidney injury requiring dialysis. JAMA 2009;302:1179–1185.

17 Clec'h C, Darmon M, Lautrette A, Chemouni F, Azoulay E, Schwebel C, et al: Efficacy of renal replacement therapy in critically ill patients: a propensity analysis. Crit Care 2012; 16:R236.

18 Bagshaw SM, Uchino S, Kellum JA, Morimatsu H, Morgera S, Schetz M, et al: Association between renal replacement therapy in critically ill patients with severe acute kidney injury and mortality. J Crit Care 2013;28: 1011–1018.

19 Kawarazaki H, Uchino S, Tokuhira N, Ohnuma T, Namba Y, Katayama S, et al: Who may not benefit from continuous renal replacement therapy in acute kidney injury? Hemodial Int 2013;17:624–632.

20 Clark EG, Bagshaw SM: Unnecessary renal replacement therapy for acute kidney injury is harmful for renal recovery. Semin Dial 2015;28:6–11.

21 Liborio AB, Leite TT, Neves FM, Teles F, Bezerra CT: AKI complications in critically ill patients: association with mortality rates and RRT. Clin J Am Soc Nephrol: CJASN 2015; 10:21–28.

22 Vaara ST, Reinikainen M, Wald R, Bagshaw SM, Pettila V, Group FS: Timing of RRT based on the presence of conventional indications. Clin J Am Soc Nephrol: CJASN 2014;9: 1577–1585.

23 Karvellas CJ, Farhat MR, Sajjad I, Mogensen SS, Leung AA, Wald R, et al: A comparison of early versus late initiation of renal replacement therapy in critically ill patients with acute kidney injury: a systematic review and meta-analysis. Crit Care 2011;15:R72.

24 Seabra VF, Balk EM, Liangos O, Sosa MA, Cendoroglo M, Jaber BL: Timing of renal replacement therapy initiation in acute renal failure: a meta-analysis. Am J Kid Dis 2008; 52:272–284.
25 Ostermann M, Dickie H, Barrett NA: Renal replacement therapy in critically ill patients with acute kidney injury – when to start. Nephrol Dial Transplant 2012;27:2242–2248.
26 Clark E, Wald R, Levin A, Bouchard J, Adhikari NK, Hladunewich M, et al: Timing the initiation of renal replacement therapy for acute kidney injury in Canadian intensive care units: a multicentre observational study. Can J Anaesth 2012;59:861–870.
27 Iyem H, Tavli M, Akcicek F, Buket S: Importance of early dialysis for acute renal failure after an open-heart surgery. Hemodial Int 2009;13:55–61.
28 Jun M, Bellomo R, Cass A, Gallagher M, Lo S, Lee J, et al: Timing of renal replacement therapy and patient outcomes in the randomized evaluation of normal versus augmented level of replacement therapy study. Crit Care Med 2014;42:1756–1765.
29 Liu KD, Himmelfarb J, Paganini E, Ikizler TA, Soroko SH, Mehta RL, et al: Timing of initiation of dialysis in critically ill patients with acute kidney injury. Clin J Am Soc Nephrol: CJASN 2006;1:915–919.
30 Shiao CC, Wu VC, Li WY, Lin YF, Hu FC, Young GH, et al: Late initiation of renal replacement therapy is associated with worse outcomes in acute kidney injury after major abdominal surgery. Crit Care 2009;13:R171.
31 Wald R, Adhikari NK, Smith OM, Weir MA, Pope K, Cohen A, et al: Comparison of standard and accelerated initiation of renal replacement therapy in acute kidney injury. Kid Int 2015;88:897–904.
32 Wald R, Bagshaw SM: The timing of renal replacement therapy initiation in acute kidney injury: is earlier truly better?*. Crit Care Med 2014;42:1933–1934.
33 Mehta RL, Pascual MT, Soroko S, Chertow GM, Group PS: Diuretics, mortality, and nonrecovery of renal function in acute renal failure. JAMA 2002;288:2547–2553.
34 Payen D, Mateo J, Cavaillon JM, Fraisse F, Floriot C, Vicaut E, et al: Impact of continuous venovenous hemofiltration on organ failure during the early phase of severe sepsis: a randomized controlled trial. Crit Care Med 2009;37:803–810.
35 Durmaz I, Yagdi T, Calkavur T, Mahmudov R, Apaydin AZ, Posacioglu H, et al: Prophylactic dialysis in patients with renal dysfunction undergoing on-pump coronary artery bypass surgery. Ann Thorac Surg 2003;75:859–864.
36 Sugahara S, Suzuki H: Early start on continuous hemodialysis therapy improves survival rate in patients with acute renal failure following coronary bypass surgery. Hemodial Int 2004;8:320–325.
37 Wang X, Jie Yuan W: Timing of initiation of renal replacement therapy in acute kidney injury: a systematic review and meta-analysis. Ren Fail 2012;34:396–402.
38 Augustine JJ, Sandy D, Seifert TH, Paganini EP: A randomized controlled trial comparing intermittent with continuous dialysis in patients with ARF. Am J Kid Dis 2004;44:1000–1007.
39 Bouman CS, Oudemans-Van Straaten HM, Tijssen JG, Zandstra DF, Kesecioglu J: Effects of early high-volume continuous venovenous hemofiltration on survival and recovery of renal function in intensive care patients with acute renal failure: a prospective, randomized trial. Crit Care Med 2002;30:2205–2211.
40 Jamale TE, Hase NK, Kulkarni M, Pradeep KJ, Keskar V, Jawale S, et al: Earlier-start versus usual-start dialysis in patients with community-acquired acute kidney injury: a randomized controlled trial. Am J Kid Dis 2013; 62:1116–1121.
41 Hamel MB, Phillips RS, Davis RB, Desbiens N, Connors AF Jr, Teno JM, et al: Outcomes and cost-effectiveness of initiating dialysis and continuing aggressive care in seriously ill hospitalized adults. SUPPORT Investigators. Study to Understand Prognoses and Preferences for Outcomes and Risks of Treatments. Ann Intern Med 1997;127:195–202.
42 Gabbay E, Meyer KB: Identifying critically ill patients with acute kidney injury for whom renal replacement therapy is inappropriate: an exercise in futility? NDT Plus 2009;2:97–103.

43 Barbar SD, Binquet C, Monchi M, Bruyere R, Quenot JP: Impact on mortality of the timing of renal replacement therapy in patients with severe acute kidney injury in septic shock: the IDEAL-ICU study (initiation of dialysis early versus delayed in the intensive care unit): study protocol for a randomized controlled trial. Trials 2014;15:270.

44 Gaudry S, Hajage D, Schortgen F, Martin-Lefevre L, Tubach F, Pons B, et al: Comparison of two strategies for initiating renal replacement therapy in the intensive care unit: study protocol for a randomized controlled trial (AKIKI). Trials 2015;16:170.

45 Conger JD: A controlled evaluation of prophylactic dialysis in post-traumatic acute renal failure. J Trauma 1975;15:1056–1063.

46 Pursnani ML, Hazra DK, Singh B, Pandey DN: Early haemodialysis in acute tubular necrosis. J Assoc Physicians India 1997;45:850–852.

Sean M. Bagshaw, MD, MSc, FRCPC
Division of Critical Care Medicine
Faculty of Medicine and Dentistry, University of Alberta
2–124E, Clinical Sciences Building, 8440-112 ST NW, Edmonton, T6G 2B7 (Canada)
E-Mail bagshaw@ualberta.ca

# Pediatric Continuous Renal Replacement Therapy

Zaccaria Ricci[a] · Stuart L. Goldstein[b]

[a]Department of Pediatric Cardiosurgery, Bambino Gesù Children's Hospital, IRCCS, Rome, Italy; [b]Center for Acute Care Nephrology, Cincinnati Children's Hospital Medical Center, Cincinnati, Ohio, USA

## Abstract

***Background:*** Continuous renal replacement therapy (CRRT) and peritoneal dialysis are the preferred forms of dialysis delivery in critically ill children for the treatment of severe acute kidney injury. The epidemiology and the outcome of acute pediatric dialysis will be reviewed. ***Summary:*** The prospective pediatric CRRT (pCRRT) registry has provided important epidemiologic information: pCRRT is required in about 5% of patients in pediatric intensive care units, and the mortality rate of these patients is about 60%. CRRT outcomes are significantly associated with age, the presence of multiple organ dysfunction syndrome and the amount of fluid overload in children before CRRT inception. The timing and the dose of pCRRT are to be further evaluated in prospective trials. A final aspect worthy of review is a technical issue: the accuracy of new-generation CRRT monitors and novel dedicated circuits that have been developed. In future years, the delivery and the outcome of pCRRT are expected to significantly improve, with the target of expanding and anticipating dialysis initiation in critically ill pediatric patients.

© 2016 S. Karger AG, Basel

## Epidemiology of Pediatric Continuous Renal Replacement Therapy

Typically, pediatric continuous renal replacement therapy (CRRT; pCRRT) is prescribed according to local expertise and without the utilization of any specific recommendation. The prospective pCRRT (ppCRRT) registry is the main source of observational information on the practice of pCRRT (in the United

States) and is currently the only reliable published report of the clinical experience derived from hundreds of treated children [1]. The ppCRRT registry was founded in 2001 and included 13 pediatric centers in the United States. Comprehensive data on 344 patients ranging from 1 day to 25 years of age and from 1.3 to 160 kg in weight are currently available; 11 different primary diagnoses were described in the registry, including sepsis, stem cell transplantation, cardiac disease, liver disease, and oncologic diagnoses [1]. The overall mortality of these patients is around 42%, but this rate is significantly higher in patients with multiple organ dysfunction syndrome and fluid overload, those weighting less than 10 kg and those receiving stem cell transplantation [1]. The ppCRRT registry also focuses on several technical aspects, such as the position and size of dialysis catheters, filter lifespan and anticoagulation. However, several issues remain controversial. (1) The optimal timing of pCRRT is a matter of ongoing debate (although it is now clear that pCRRT should be considered before fluid accumulates in children). (2) The dose and the level of adequate dialytic delivery in children (including the significant differences between neonates and older children) remain to be established. (3) The long-term outcomes of acute kidney injury (AKI) children undergoing CRRT need urgent analysis because emerging evidence indicates that patients surviving CRRT often have reduced renal reserve and do not achieve restoration of premorbid renal function.

**Timing**

Studies on the timing of pCRRT are difficult; in general, retrospective or post hoc analyses investigated the issue of timing, but the lack of absolute indications for dialysis inception contributed to the absence of a common definition of 'timing'. This limitation has significantly hampered the search for a definitive answer to the question of adequate timing. As a common sense rule, 'timely' CRRT initiation has been supported by several authors [2]. According to the current evidence, it might be reasonable to suggest that pCRRT be instituted rapidly in oligoanuric patients, especially in patients with significant fluid accumulation, before the fluid overload threshold of 10–20% has been reached [3]. An interesting post hoc analysis of the Randomized Evaluation of Normal versus Augmented Level Replacement Therapy (RENAL) trial clearly showed that the mortality rate of adult patients undergoing CRRT was affected by the level of fluid balance achieved after the initial 48 hours of therapy [4]. A similar but small retrospective observational study of pCRRT patients undergoing extracorporeal membrane oxygenation (ECMO) showed that survival is associated with the level of fluid overload at the time of CRRT initiation and that 'forcing' fluid removal in order to improve patient outcomes may be reasonable [5]. By defining pCRRT timing as the interval from intensive care unit (ICU) admission to CRRT initiation, the authors of a large retrospective 10-year cohort study [6] found that late initiators (>5 days after ICU admission) had a higher mortality rate than early initiators (≤5 days after ICU admission), with a hazard ratio of 1.56 (95% confidence interval: 1.02–2.37) and an increase of 5% in mortality for every day of delay in CRRT initiation after adjusting for significant confounders. Based on multivariate regression analysis, independent predictors of mortality included fluid overload, indication for CRRT initiation (simultaneous presence of renal dysfunction and fluid overload), severity of illness at ICU admission and active oncologic diagnosis. Interestingly, according to the pediatric modified risk, injury, failure, loss, and end stage (pRIFLE) classification, the authors seemed to realize that many severe cases at ICU admission were more likely to be treated earlier (hence, patients categorized into the most severe pRIFLE classes were more common in the survivor group). Conversely, if a patient slowly but significantly progressed to higher AKI stages during the course of the ICU stay, treatment was delayed; as a result, a correlation between pRIFLE class progression and time to CRRT initiation was found. It is possible that this subgroup of patients may receive the most benefit from earlier CRRT initiation. If a patient has AKI, pCRRT has to be started within 5 days of ICU admission in order to be effective in terms of mortality [6].

**Continuous Renal Replacement Therapy Modalities**

Peritoneal dialysis (PD) and CRRT are the most frequently used modalities in infants to date. PD is generally applied to neonates, unless specific contraindications are present (i.e. peritonitis, abdominal masses or bleeding) [7]. PD uses the peritoneum as a semi-permeable membrane to achieve solute diffusion and plasma water ultrafiltration; a dialysate is infused through an abdominal catheter, and after a period of so-called 'dwell time', waste solution is drained from the abdomen. Typically, in order to avoid excessive increases in intra-abdominal pressure during dialysis, especially in high-risk patients (i.e. post-cardiac surgery), a 'low flow' prescription of 10 ml/kg dialysate is delivered [8]. This approach is also useful for preventing hemodynamic instability secondary to reduced venous return caused by inferior vena cava compression. Dwell times may vary from 10 to 30 minutes according to the needed dose. As a general rule, dialysate tonicity (based on the glucose concentration, 1.36–2.5%) is responsible for peritoneal net ultrafiltration. PD is simple and safe, and it can be administered without dedicated technology. Moreover, a steep learning curve is not needed: PD is typically administered by ICU nurses without specific expertise in dialysis. Nonetheless, PD is certainly limited by a lack of efficiency; water removal appears to be particularly difficult in selected patients, and this is a major issue in patients with severe fluid overload. Other important flaws of PD use are the possibilities of interstitial fluid accumulation in cases of suboptimal dialysate drainage, hyperglycemia and peritoneal infection. PD is obviously contraindicated in patients with recent abdominal surgery or abdominal bleeding [7]. As a matter of fact, PD is frequently applied to post-cardiac surgery patients, and its main advantage is its availability to be started in a very early phase of oligo-anuria or fluid retention. PD has recently been shown to be associated with improved survival in a large cohort of post-cardiac surgery neonates receiving PD within the first 24 post-operative hours compared with patients who received PD beyond the second post-operative day [9].

As an alternative to PD, extracorporeal dialysis in children can be conducted together with intermittent hemodialysis and CRRT: these therapies can theoretically be delivered as hemofiltration, hemodialysis or hemodiafiltration [10]. The choice of dialysis modality may be influenced by several factors, including local expertise and preferences, the required dialytic targets, and the clinical profile of the treated baby. Intermittent dialysis may not be well tolerated in hemodynamically unstable critically ill infants because of a rapid rate of solute clearance and net fluid removal. These children are generally treated via CRRT, which reasonably removes fluid and solutes, including pro-inflammatory mediators. Circuits with reduced priming volume together with monitors that provide extremely accurate fluid balance are still not commercially available [10]. The current literature, however, has focused on the possibility of treating fluid overload in patients at the start of dialysis. It is clearly established that at the time of dialysis initiation, survivors tend to have less fluid overload than nonsurvivors, especially in the setting of multiple organ dysfunction syndrome [11]. In contrast to the observations in adult patients, in whom dialysis dose may play a key role in outcome, in small children, adequate water content is the main independent predictor of outcome.

With regard to the CRRT modality, solute clearance resulting from the three different modes of CRRT at the low blood flow rates typically used in pediatric patients were compared; postdilution continuous venovenous hemofiltration (CVVH) and continuous venovenous hemodialysis gave nearly equivalent clearances [12]. At the low blood flow rates used in pediatric patients, which raise concerns that the high filtration fractions during postdilution CVVH may cause excessive hemoconcentration and filter clotting, continuous venovenous hemodialysis appeared to be the optimal modality for maximizing clearance of small solutes during CRRT. Nevertheless, the following advantage of hemofiltration compared to hemodialysis should be taken in consideration: medium and high molecular weight solutes are significantly more effectively removed by convective modalities [13]. In light of these considerations, predilution hemofiltration might be the preferred modality for pediatric patients. To date, there have been no randomized trials guiding the prescription of CRRT in children. A small solute clearance of 2 l/h*1.73 m$^2$ may be recommended, and this rate is typically utilized in the United States [14]. It must be noted that such a prescription may lead to a significantly higher dialytic dose if applied in proportion to the dose in adult patients and that the advantages of high-intensity treatments have to be calibrated with the risk of unnecessary removal of useful plasma elements (e.g. antibodies, amino acids, and brain natriuretic peptide) [15]. Figure 1 provides a tentative approach to modality selection for pediatric patients.

## Technical Aspects of Pediatric Continuous Renal Replacement Therapy

During the last decade, CRRT technology has significantly improved. We are currently facing the release of the fourth generation of dialytic monitors into the market. These monitors are equipped with multiple safety features and control algorithms, as well as extremely accurate pumps and scales; as a matter of fact, 'standard' CRRT is a safe practice today [16]. However, pCRRT cannot be considered as a part of 'standard' care. In some cases, CRRT machines designed for adults have been equipped with pediatric circuits and lines in an attempt to comply with the specific requirements of very small patients. With this detail in mind, we can reasonably state that most, if not all, machines are currently used off-label in patients below 10 kg. This is mainly due to the small number of pediatric cases, which has ultimately resulted in a limited interest of industry in developing a fully dedicated device for small children. Furthermore, manufacturers of dialysis or CRRT machines do not perform specific tests for treatments in patients smaller than 10–15 kg, and safety features are not specifically created for these patients; legal concerns may arise when operators decide to prescribe these therapies to small children. In current practice, the clinical application of dialysis equipment to pediatric patients is substantially adapted to smaller patients despite great concerns about the outcomes and the side effects of such extracorporeal therapies. Under these conditions, smaller patients do not rely on the same extremely accurate delivery of therapy as that received by adults, especially concerning fluid balance. In this context, the Cardio-Renal Pediatric Dialysis Emergency Machine (CARPEDIEM) was designed in Vicenza in 2011 in order to provide the basis for the development of renal replacement therapy (RRT) equipment specifically dedicated to newborns and small infants with a

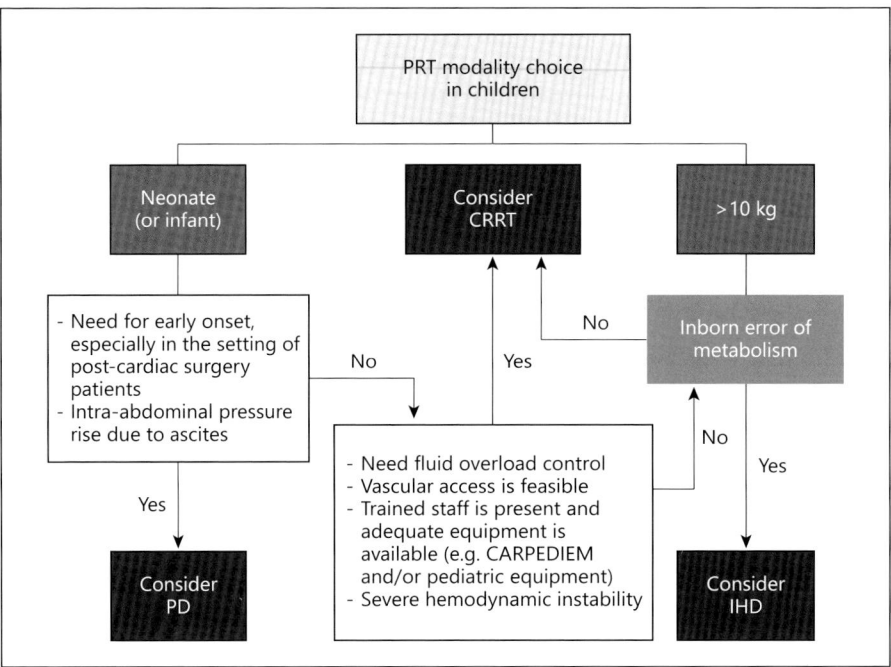

**Fig. 1.** The first step in deciding whether to prescribe continuous renal replacement therapy to pediatric patients is an evaluation of the patient's age (or weight); in the case of small babies (below 10 kg), peritoneal dialysis might be considered as an option. Peritoneal dialysis is particularly recommended in post-cardiac surgery patients who need an early onset of renal replacement therapy or in patients who are experiencing increased intra-abdominal pressure due to ascites. If such a patient requires fluid overload control due to significant fluid overload (>20%) or if his/her critical state includes severe hemodynamic instability, extracorporeal continuous renal replacement therapy (CRRT) might be the most appropriate renal replacement therapy. Other important requirements for CRRT delivery are the presence of adequate vascular access and the availability of CRRT equipment. All other pediatric critically ill patients who do not require dialysis due to an inborn error of metabolism (i.e. hyperammonemia) should be treated with CRRT, provided that dedicated pediatric equipment and adequately accurate dialytic monitors are available.

weight range of 2.0–9.9 kg and with an approximate body surface area from 0.15 to 0.5 m$^2$. In these patients, the total blood volume ranges from less than 200 ml to about 1 liter, meaning that total body water content varies from 1 to 5 liters. In such cases, the priming volumes of dialysis circuits should be reduced to a minimum level, and roller pumps should be run at a slow speed to maintain a good level of accuracy and to ensure line integrity (small roller pumps running small tubes are expected to quickly decline in performance) [17]. The first patients are currently being treated, and relevant results have recently been published [18]. As a confirmation of the growing interest in research in this field, another pediatric monitor for continuous dialysis, the Newcastle infant dialysis and ultrafiltration system (Nidus) has been recently described. The Nidus [19] is an original machine driven by syringes instead of roller pumps, providing single-needle vascular access. The circuit volume of the Nidus is only 13 ml, and very interestingly, there is no need for circuit blood-priming. Recently, Coulthard and coworkers treated 10 babies weighing between 1.8 and 5.9 kg and reported satisfactory machine performance with respect to the adequacy of clearance and machine accuracy [19]. Further studies of these two interesting devices are warranted, and a significant outcome improvement for neonates with severe AKI requiring RRT may be expected from these innovations.

## Continuous Renal Replacement Therapy in Extracorporeal Membrane Oxygenation Patients

With the recent increase in the complexity of critically ill patients, in high resource centers, a peculiar category of AKI patient is one who requires both RRT and ECMO; such patients are frequently seen in the pediatric setting because the vast majority of children receiving ECMO exhibit severe renal injury, especially after severe cardiac dysfunction (cardio-renal syndrome) or aggressive mechanical ventilation (lung-renal syndrome). The CRRT circuit may be placed in parallel (blood flow running in the same direction as the ECMO circuit) or in series (blood flow running countercurrent to the ECMO circuit). Santiago and coauthors described how to connect the CRRT device into the ECMO circuit [20]: the inlet (arterial) line of the CRRT circuit was connected after the ECMO blood pump using a three-way stopcock that was also used for the infusion of heparin, and the outlet (venous) line was connected to the circuit at another stopcock before the oxygenator. Alternatively to the suggestion by the authors, the inlet of the CRRT machine may be connected after the ECMO pump and the filter outlet and then returned to the ECMO circuit before the pump (into the reservoir, if present). A CRRT circuit running countercurrent to extracorporeal assistance allows the blood treated via RRT to be aspirated from the arterial ECMO section (where blood returns to the patient) and then be infused into the venous ECMO section (where the patient is drained) [21]. This alternative set-up might reduce blood flow resistance and turbulence after the centrifugal pump and might improve reservoir drainage when a roller pump is present. The blood recirculation induced by these circuit set-ups is negligible, considering that the CRRT to ECMO blood flow ratio is never greater than 0.1. Dr. Shaheen et al. [22] presented their experience with two different subgroups of children: one group that required hemofiltration alone and another group that required hemofiltration and ECMO. Not surprisingly, the authors identified a higher mortality rate in patients requiring CVVH and ECMO than in patients requiring hemofiltration alone. The authors proposed that certain therapies should be reserved for experienced teams. Performing CVVH in a heterogeneous population with large age and weight ranges poses significant clinical and technical challenges. The low frequency of CVVH use in combination with ECMO, as well as the use of other extracorporeal therapies, also raises problems with maintaining nursing skills. Objective clinical and biochemical markers for commencing CVVH alone or in combination with ECMO remain to be defined. Several studies, however, already showed the safety and feasibility of this combined therapy in a pediatric setting [23]; although some concerns about this difficult combined therapy have been raised (i.e. fluid balance accuracy [24]), the application of CRRT to all patients receiving ECMO is indeed currently recommended by some authors [25, 26]. In a matched control study, 15 newborns receiving ECMO in combination with continuous hemofiltration were compared with 46 historical controls. The times on extracorporeal assistance and on mechanical ventilation were significantly reduced in the CRRT population. Therefore, such a strategy might improve fluid balance management and alleviate capillary leak syndrome. Furthermore, according to these authors, fewer blood transfusions are needed, and the overall cost per ECMO run is lower.

**Conclusion**

Severe AKI requiring RRT is a severe clinical condition that results in the death of more than 50% of treated patients, and dialyzing critically ill children is further complicated by several technical issues. Early diagnosis, prevention, conservative measures and novel technology are all part of a multidimensional approach to dialytic adequacy in critically ill children. The outcomes of dialysis may vary significantly depending on the underlying disease, the severity of illness, the time of intervention and the institutional expertise and practices. Several aspects, primarily including pCRRT timing, still require significant research and have great uncertainty. So far, the outcomes of critically ill children requiring CRRT are poor, and a strategy for improvement is urgently needed. The long-term outcomes of survivors, especially those who do not completely recover baseline function and younger patients, are potentially hampered by chronic renal dysfunction. In this scenario, new technological advances, such as miniaturized circuits and membranes, accurate CRRT machines and effective prescription schedules, hold promise for assisting the clinician in improving treatment quality.

## References

1 Sutherland SM, Goldstein SL, Alexander SR: The Prospective Pediatric Continuous Renal Replacement Therapy (ppCRRT) registry: a critical appraisal. Pediatr Nephrol 2014;29: 2069–2076.
2 Ricci Z, Ronco C: Timing, dose and mode of dialysis in acute kidney injury. Curr Opin Crit Care 2011;17:556–561.
3 Sutherland SM, Zappitelli M, Alexander SR, et al: Fluid overload and mortality in children receiving continuous renal replacement therapy: the prospective pediatric continuous renal replacement therapy registry. Am J Kidney Dis 2010;55:316–325.
4 The RENAL Replacement Therapy Study Investigators. An observational study fluid balance and patient outcomes in the randomized evaluation of normal vs augmented level of replacement therapy trial. Crit Care Med 2012;40:1753–1760.
5 Selewski DT, Cornell TT, Blatt NB, et al: Fluid overload and fluid removal in pediatric patients on extracorporeal membrane oxygenation requiring continuous renal replacement therapy. Crit Care Med 2012;40:2694–2699.
6 Modem V, Thompson M, Gollhofer D, et al: Timing of continuous renal replacement therapy and mortality in critically ill children. Crit Care Med 2014;42:943–953.
7 Morelli S, Ricci Z, Di Chiara L, et al: Renal replacement therapy in neonates with congenital heart disease. Contrib Nephrol 2007; 156:428–433.
8 Ricci Z, Morelli S, Ronco C, et al: Inotropic support and peritoneal dialysis adequacy in neonates after cardiac surgery. Interact Cardiovasc Thorac Surg 2008;7:116–120.
9 Bojan M, Gioanni S, Vouhé PR, et al: Early initiation of peritoneal dialysis in neonates and infants with acute kidney injury following cardiac surgery is associated with a significant decrease in mortality. Kidney Int 2012;82:474–481.
10 Picca S, Ricci Z, Picardo S: Acute kidney injury in an infant after cardiopulmonary bypass. Semin Nephrol. 2008;28:470–476.
11 Goldstein SL, Somers MJ, Baum MA, et al: Pediatric patients with multi-organ dysfunction syndrome receiving continuous renal replacement therapy. Kidney Int 2005;67: 653–658.
12 Parakininkas D, Greenbaum LA: Comparison of solute clearance in three modes of continuous renal replacement therapy. Pediatr Crit Care Med 2004;5:269–274.
13 Ricci Z, Ronco C, Bachetoni A, et al: Solute removal during continuous renal replacement therapy in critically ill patients: convection versus diffusion. Crit Care 2006;10:R67.
14 Askenazi DJ, Goldstein SL, Koralkar R, et al: Continuous renal replacement therapy for children ≤10 kg: a report from the prospective pediatric continuous renal replacement therapy registry. J Pediatr 2013;162:587–592. e3.
15 Maynar Moliner J, Honore PM, Sánchez-Izquierdo Riera JA, et al: Handling continuous renal replacement therapy-related adverse effects in intensive care unit patients: the dialytrauma concept. Blood Purif 2012;34:177–185.
16 Wald R, Adhikari NK, Smith OM, et al: Comparison of standard and accelerated initiation of renal replacement therapy in acute kidney injury. Kidney Int 2015;88:897–904.
17 Ronco C, Garzotto F, Ricci Z: CA.R.PE. DI.E.M. (Cardio-Renal Pediatric Dialysis Emergency Machine): evolution of continuous renal replacement therapies in infants. A personal journey. Pediatr Nephrol 2012;27: 1203–1211.
18 Ronco C, Garzotto F, Brendolan A, et al: Continuous renal replacement therapy in neonates and small infants: development and first-in-human use of a miniaturised machine (CARPEDIEM). Lancet 2014;383:1807–1813.
19 Coulthard MG, Crosier J, Griffiths C, et al: Haemodialysing babies weighing <8 kg with the Newcastle infant dialysis and ultrafiltration system (Nidus): comparison with peritoneal and conventional haemodialysis. Pediatr Nephrol 2014;29:1873–1881.
20 Santiago MJ, Sánchez A, López-Herce J, et al: The use of continuous renal replacement therapy in series with extracorporeal membrane oxygenation. Kidney Int 2009;76:1289–1292.
21 Ricci Z, Ronco C, Picardo S. CRRT in series with extracorporeal membrane oxygenation in pediatric patients. Kidney Int 2010;77: 469–470.

22 Shaheen IS, Harvey B, Watson AR, et al: Continuous venovenous hemofiltration with or without extracorporeal membrane oxygenation in children. Pediatr Crit Care Med 2007;8:362–365.
23 Symons JM, McMahon MW, Karamlou T, et al: Continuous renal replacement therapy with an automated monitor is superior to a free-flow system during extracorporeal life support. Pediatr Crit Care Med 2013;14: e404–e408.
24 Ricci Z, Morelli S, Vitale V, et al: Management of fluid balance in continuous renal replacement therapy: technical evaluation in the pediatric setting. Int J Artif Organs 2007; 30:896–901.
25 Hoover NG, Heard M, Reid C, et al: Enhanced fluid management with continuous venovenous hemofiltration in pediatric respiratory failure patients receiving extracorporeal membrane oxygenation support. Intensive Care Med 2008;34:2241–2247.
26 Blijdorp K, Cransberg K, Wildschut ED, et al: Haemofiltration in newborns treated with extracorporeal membrane oxygenation: a case-comparison study. Crit Care 2009;13: R48.

Zaccaria Ricci
Department of Pediatric Cardiosurgery, Bambino Gesù Children's Hospital, IRCCS
Piazza S. Onofrio 400165
IT–00100 Rome (Italy)
E-Mail z.ricci@libero.it

Stuart L. Goldstein, MD
Center for Acute Care Nephrology, Cincinnati Children's Hospital Medical Center
3333 Burnet Avenue, MLC 7022
Cincinnati, OH 45206 (USA)
E-Mail stuart.goldstein@cchmc.org

# Management of Cardiac Surgery-Associated Acute Kidney Injury

Jiarui Xu[a–d] · Wuhua Jiang[a–d] · Yi Fang[a–d] · Jie Teng[a–d] · Xiaoqiang Ding[a–d]

[a]Division of Nephrology, Zhongshan Hospital, Shanghai Medical College, Fudan University, [b]Shanghai Institute for Kidney and Dialysis, [c]Key Laboratory of Kidney and Blood Purification of Shanghai, [d]Quality Control Center of Dialysis, Shanghai, China

## Abstract

Cardiac surgery-associated acute kidney injury (CSA-AKI) is known to be a common complication of cardiac surgery that is associated with poor short- and long-term outcomes. The causes of CSA-AKI include the discovered or undiscovered risk factors within the perioperative course, mostly non-modifiable; some are even iatrogenic. Recognizing and mediating risk factors preoperatively and optimizing intraoperative practices may decrease the incidence of CSA-AKI. By now, the present studies cannot confirm which drugs are better off for preventing CSA-AKI. The effect and whether early administration of these drugs to prevent CSA-AKI is effective remain uncertain, so is the administration of renal replacement therapy. We will demonstrate some typical studies that focus on the prevention of CSA-AKI and may delight further research.     © 2016 S. Karger AG, Basel

## Definition of CSA-AKI

With the rising acknowledgment and update of definition in AKI, the incidence of CSA-AKI ranges between 8.9 and 39% [1, 2]. And about 1–5% developed severe AKI for which renal replacement therapy (RRT) was needed [3]. The consensus definitions of AKI were based on 1.5- to 2-fold increases in serum creatinine (SCr) [4]. Such traditional definitions of AKI have not been considered sensitive enough for the severity of renal injury that may be detected by subtle elevations in SCr such as those used by the Acute Kidney Injury Network (AKIN) and Risk, Injury, Failure, Loss, End-stage renal disease (RIFLE) definitions. These two criteria were compared, and both were proven to be accurate and

**Table 1.** Biomarkers that have been clinically investigated

| Biomarker | Origin in nephron |
|---|---|
| NGAL | Glomerulus, distal tubule, collecting duct |
| Cystatin C | Glomerulus, proximal tubule |
| Interleukin-18 | Proximal tubule |
| KIM-1 | Proximal tubule |
| L-FABP | Proximal tubule |
| NAG | Proximal tubule, distal tubule |
| Urine αGST | Proximal tubule |
| Urine βGST | Distal tubule |
| Netrin-1 | Proximal tubule |
| Hepcidin | Proximal tubule |
| Urinary calprotectin | Collecting duct |
| TIMP-2 | Proximal tubule |
| IGFBP7 | Proximal tubule |
| TLR 3 | Proximal tubule |
| β2-microglobulin | Glomerulus |

GST = Glutathione S-transferase; IGFBP7 = insulin-like growth factor-binding protein 7; KIM-1 = kidney injury molecule-1; L-FABP = liver-type fatty acid-binding protein; NAG = N-acetyl-β-D-glucosaminidase; NGAL = neutrophil gelatinase-associated lipocalin; TIMP-2 = tissue inhibitor of metalloproteinases-2; TLR 3 = toll-like receptor 3.

early predictors of mortality [5]. In 2012, the Kidney Disease: Improving Global Outcomes (KDIGO) Workgroup produced clinical guidelines for AKI that was meant to supplement AKIN and RIFLE classifications [6]. But none of the present criteria can identify AKI at the right time of renal injury yet.

Many biomarkers have been studied but very few have been used clinically. Some biomarkers were proved applicable in small single-center trials, but they shall need to be proved in a larger scale or races also. In the future, research on these biomarkers will surely improve the outcome in patients (table 1) [7]. Validated consensus definitions of AKI including biomarkers should be developed to predict milder AKI.

**Prevention of CSA-AKI**

Knowing risk factors that cause CSA-AKI may help to create strategies to prevent AKI in the preoperative and intraoperative phases of care. Furthermore, management of some modifiable factors such as anemia, cardiopulmonary bypass (CPB) duration, perioperative red blood cell (RBC) transfusions and contrast media insult may also be effective.

**Table 2.** Risk factors for CSA-AKI [8]

*Non-modifiable*
Old age
Male sex
Black race
Pre-existing chronic kidney disease
Proteinuria or elevated albumin-to-creatinine ratio
Hypertension
Diabetes mellitus
Chronic liver disease and/or complications of portal hypertension
Heart failure and/or decreased ejection fraction
Coronary artery disease and/or recent myocardial infarction
Chronic obstructive pulmonary disease
Peripheral vascular disease
Malignancy

*Potentially modifiable*
Anemia
Critical illness
Sepsis
Trauma
Cardiac surgery
Major non-cardiac surgery
Exposure to radiocontrast media
Fluid overload
Fluid resuscitation with synthetic colloids (hydroxyethyl starch) or chloride rich solutions (0.9% saline)
Drug toxicity, drug interactions or nephrotoxic medications
High-risk or emergency procedures

*Risk Factors*

Risk factors (table 2) for CSA-AKI include non-modifiable and potentially modifiable factors [8]. The results may incorporate extended intensive care unit (ICU) stay, hospital stay, increased need for short- and long-term RRTs, progression of chronic kidney disease (CKD) and increased short- and long-term mortalities.

*Optimizing Surgical Procedure*

The application of CPB was regarded as an important risk factor of CSA-AKI. The bio-incompatibility of the artificial CPB set was known to be the most likely reason. Of course, there are some methods to strengthen the biocompatibility of the CPB set, for instance, coating the phosphorylcholine. Since CPB is one such cause leading to CSA-AKI, some surgical doctors are getting interested in the off-pump coronary artery bypass (OPCAB), which was applied to alleviate CPB-related complications, including CSA-AKI. With this procedure, renal perfusion can be improved, and other severe complications, such as SIRS can be avoided. The incidence of CSA-AKI can also be reduced by OPCAB, so as to the length of stay. A large sample observational study concluded that in CKD patients who went through the OPCAB, the incidence of RRT was lower than in those who went through coronary artery bypass grafting (CABG) with CPB application [9]. Another meta-analysis incorporated 22 randomize controlled trials and concluded less incidence of CSA-AKI in the OPCAB population than in those who underwent CABG [10].

*Avoidance of Transfusions*

Anemia is common in patients being treated with cardiac surgery, especially preoperative. Preoperative anemia was one independent risk factor for CSA-AKI [2]. But unfortunately, there was always not enough time to assess the degree of anemia, not even to treat anemia before cardiac surgery or catheterization. So perioperative transfusion has been inevitable to most anemia patients. Transfusion of erythrocyte can improve organ function by increasing oxygen delivery. But many studies have concluded that erythrocyte transfusion may result in severe complications, especially CSA-AKI, leading to organ injury. This may be due to the increase of tissue oxidative stress and the activated coagulation cascade [2].

*Contrast Media Insult*

Patients often receive cardiac surgery after coronary angiography during the same admission day because of their poor instability status and threatening anatomy as well as non-urgent reasons such as patient or provider convenience. Iodinated contrast material causes a series of vasodilatations that may contribute to intrarenal vasoconstriction and ischemic injury known as contrast-induced acute kidney injury (CI-AKI). The rise in creatinine may occur up to 48 h after the injury. So when coronary angiography and cardiac surgery occur during the same hospitalization, there is an increased risk for AKI. Extension of the interval between the two procedures as coronary angiography with discharge and readmission for the surgery is necessary.

KDIGO recommend using either iso-osmolar or low-osmolar iodinated contrast media, rather than high-osmolar iodinated contrast media (1B), and intravenous volume expansion with either isotonic sodium chloride or sodium bicarbonate solutions, rather than no intravenous volume expansion, in patients at increased risk for CI-AKI (1A). Besides these approaches, many studies have shown that N-Acetylcysteine (NAC) may prevent CI-AKI. A meta-analysis showed that a combination of NAC with prophylaxis and sodium bicarbonate reduced the occurrence of CI-AKI by 35% and should be strongly suggested for all high-risk patients [11]. KDIGO also recommend using oral NAC, together with intravenous isotonic crystalloids to prevent AKI (2D) [6].

## Therapeutic Interventions in CSA-AKI

*Drugs*
A number of drug therapies have been studied as potential preventive agents for CSA-AKI. Controversies remain on them because trials in different centers often showed different results.

*Statins*
Preoperative statins have been found renoprotective through their anti-inflammatory capacity and endothelin secretion reduction. But most studies were on animals or retrospective. In a meta-analysis, the conclusion was that preoperative statins were managed in cardiac surgery and the improvement of all-cause mortality was significant [12]. Meanwhile early postoperative statin has also been found capable of reducing the incidence of CSA-AKI [13]. But the overall effect of perioperative statin application remains controversial since some studies did not conclude similar results [13, 14]. So, larger sample trials should be necessary for validating the effect on CSA-AKI reduction.

*N-Acetylcysteine*
As was mentioned above, some studies showed that NAC has the capacity of renal protection against CI-AKI [15], but the evidence is uncertain, so the application of NAC is not consensus suggested. Since the NAC protects kidney with its antioxidant capacity, some studies [16] focused on its protection against CSA-AKI.

But another meta-analyses [17] does not support their beneficial effect on the prevention of CSA-AKI. The main controversy is the dose of the drug. Some studies based on small sample RCT concluded the incidence of CSA-AKI lower in CKD stage 3–4 patients who received NAC (150 mg/kg, then 50 mg/kg infusion over 6 h) than in the control group [18]. They also found that the possible mechanism of the protective effect comes from its constraining increase in reactive oxidative species. Thus, interestingly, it is linked to the CPB once more. In this study, the morbidity of AKI in those who had CPB but did not receive NAC was 63%, much higher than those who received NAC and had OPCAB surgery (8%). This also attributed to the multifactorial CSA-AKI.

*Sodium Bicarbonate*
Sodium bicarbonate also has been studied as a potential preventive agent in CI-AKI with the mechanism as the reduction in tubular oxidative stress [19]. Urinary alkalinization has also been evaluated as a possible protective intervention

in cardiac surgery, but results of trials have been controversial. A meta-analysis concluded that combination prophylaxis with NAC and sodium bicarbonate substantially can reduce the incidence of CI-AKI by 35% and should be strongly recommended for all high-risk patients [20]. But for cardiac surgery, Tian et al. [21] performed another meta-analysis that included five RCTs and one prospective observational cohort study about sodium bicarbonate. There was no difference in the incidence of CSA-AKI.

*Fenoldopam*

The mechanism of CSA-AKI is multifactorial, for which the ischemia in the medulla is known to be the main cause. Fenoldopam is a selective agonist of dopamine-1 (DA1) receptors, and its renoprotection attributes to the vasodilation of renal vessel, mesenteric vessel, peripheral vessel and coronary artery. It is different from dopamine in that fenoldopam does not influent dopamine-2 (DA2) receptors. Thus, theoretically the vascular dilation in medulla is better than in the cortex. In one study, an adequate dose of fenoldopam was found to be beneficial for renal protection after cardiac surgery [22]. Meanwhile, some authors found the complication of hypotension after it had been administered following cardiac surgery, some patients even received vasopressors and its effect of reduction of RRT and improvement of survival and length of stay were not significantly concluded [23, 24]. According to its renal protective mechanism, fenoldopam should be studied in a lager, multicenter and powered trials to confirm its benefit and complications, and the dose should be adjusted fairly carefully to prevent its adverse effect on cardiac surgery patients.

*Renal Replacement Therapy*

RRT is still the cornerstone for the therapy of AKI after cardiac surgery. Over the years, the indications and mortality have changed a lot. But still some unresolved issues have remained as to the choosing of modality, when to start and stop, prescription for dose and fluid balance, how to achieve the adequacy of treatment, etc.

*Timing*

The general indications of emergent RRT always include life-threatening changes like the following: fluid overload, hyperkalemia, severe metabolic acidosis, severe congestive heart failure, pulmonary edema and overt symptom caused by uremia. But the timing of initiation of RRT in CSA-AKI still remains controversial. Earlier RRT initiation was concluded beneficial from previous studies that aim to remove redundant fluid or toxin in the body, correct the hyperkalemia and acidosis, stabilize the internal environment, ensure the intake of antibiotics, calorie, protein or other nutrition. Also, some studies have found that early treatment can lead to better improvement of renal function after AKI. Although the patients who have undergone RRT may have better outcome, the mortality rate has not changed much over the past 10 years [25].

In fact, the mechanism of CSA-AKI is quite different from the other cause of AKI. The relationship of pathophysiology between heart and renal is very complex and susceptible. Hemodynamic parameters include cardiac output, oxygen delivery, central venous pressure (CVP), mean arterial pressure (MAP), peripheral circulation and so on can influence the renal blood, which determines the extent of renal damage and renal outcome. So it is possible that the application of conventional indications of RRT can be more accurate and further investigations about newer indications are needed. The indications of RRT in developing countries also should include the assessment of the family, including their understanding of the severity of the primary disease or the economic situation of the family.

*Modality*

Different forms of RRT such as intermittent hemodialysis (IHD), continuous RRT (CRRT) or hybrid forms are now available for application in cardiac surgery patients. KDIGO guideline suggests using continuous and intermittent RRT as complementary therapies in AKI patients (not graded), and CRRT in hemodynamically unstable patients rather than standard intermittent RRT (grade 2B) [6]. CRRT now has become a routine therapy in many countries and IHD may suit patients during transition to RRT withdrawal or those who are ready to be moved out of ICU. In reference to some previous RCTs, there was not enough evidence for CRRT to reduce the overall mortality more significantly than IHD. But CRRT was concluded to be associated with better renal recovery compared with IHD in some systematic analysis [26].

CRRT may not be prevalent in some resource-limited places where the hybrid form which is now called prolonged intermittent RRT (PIRRT), including sustained low-efficiency (daily) dialysis (SLE(D)D) and extended daily dialysis (EDD) etc., may often be chosen. In these approaches, treatment duration ranged from 8 to 10 h and may be performed on daily basis or at least on alternate days, which can provide longer session durations with lower flows and efficiency. Randomized trial has demonstrated that switching from CRRT to PIRRT was not associated with a change in mortality rate that provides evidence that PIRRT might be equivalent to CRRT in the general ICU patient [27].

For all, the choice of modality may be including multiple aspects: efficacy, safety and feasibility. Sometimes the consideration of costs, operators or techniques may be more important.

*Dose*

Some previous studies have indicated that higher dose of RRT may benefit the patients. But two large multicenter RCT, RENAL and ATN, studies showed that increased intensity of RRT was not associated with improved outcomes [28, 29]. KDIGO guidelines recommend delivering a Kt/V of 3.9 per week when using intermittent or extended RRT in AKI (1A) or delivering an effluent volume of 20–25 ml/kg/h for CRRT in AKI (1A) [6].

It is likely an area of the dose–response relationship that may exist. Delivery of doses lower than 20 ml/kg/h should be avoided; also above a delivered RRT intensity of ~45 ml/kg/h may be associated with worse outcome. Many factors contribute to delivering a RRT dose lower than prescribed, and it is the delivered dose that is likely to affect the clinical outcome. Clotting and clinical problems represent the most common causes of treatment interruption in patients on CRRT, and such interruptions lead to large variability of administered doses. It has been shown that the delivered dialysis dose is generally lower than prescribed, ranging from 68 to 89% of prescribed, which suggests the need to prescribe about 20% more than the target [30]. To ensure outcomes similar to those seen in the ATN and RENAL trials, clinicians should also prescribe CRRT on the basis of patient body weight to the established effluent flow rate target of about 25–35 ml/kg/h.

*Ceasing Time*

Very few studies about timing of RRT withdrawal existed. KDIGO guidelines suggest discontinuing RRT when it is no longer required, either because intrinsic kidney function has recovered to the point that it is adequate to meet patient needs or because RRT is no longer consistent with the goals of care (not graded) [6]. Diuretics are not suggested to enhance kidney function recovery or to reduce the duration or frequency of RRT (2B) [6]. Assessment of kidney function in consistency with the goals of therapy for the patient is required every day. Furthermore, the discontinuation of RRT may not occur suddenly, which includes changes of modality, frequency or duration of RRT. Until now, no research or guidance is available be used to manage this process.

*GDRRT*

There are no clear evidences in optimal RRT dose and modality; the concept of goal-directed RRT (GDRRT) may be worth considering. The idea of goal directed therapy (GDT) for critically ill patients was first raised in 1973, and various GDTs have been developed to achieve hemodynamic stability during and after cardiac surgery. The concept of a GDRRT was first proposed by Mehta et al. [31], which sets the goals before RRT, then adjusts the dose, mode,

**Table 3.** The goals of GDRRT

| | |
|---|---|
| Solute | BUN ≤30 mmol/l |
| Volume | Urine output ≥0.5 ml/kg/h; 24 h fluid output ≥24 h fluid intake in volume overload patients; controlled acute pulmonary edema; reduction of peripheral edema; hematocrit ≥30% |
| Electrolyte and pH | Electrolyte and acid-base parameters normal or near normal: 3.5< potassium ≤5.5 mmol; 7.25≤ pH <7.45 |
| Hemodynamics | MAP ≥65 mm Hg without large vasoactive drugs; CVP ≥8–12 mm Hg; $SaO_2$ ≥93% |

BUN = Blood urea nitrogen; MAP = mean arterial pressure; CVP = central venous pressure; $SaO_2$ = saturation level of oxygen in hemoglobin.

anticoagulation methods, component of dialysis or replacement fluid and assistant therapies according to the goals during the treatment sessions.

We recently compared the efficacies of GDRRT and daily hemofiltration (DHF) for treating AKI patients after cardiac surgery [32]. GDRRT is composed of almost all kinds of RRT modes including hemodialysis (HD), hemofiltration (HF), ultrafiltration (UF) and hemodiafiltration (HDF). The modality, dose, duration of RRT sessions and frequency were all adjusted at any time depending on whether the goals of treatment were achieved (table 3; figure 1). Though there are no statistically significant differences in in-hospital and 30-day mortality rates, the GDRRT approach is superior in improving renal recovery, as well as in reducing the time and cost of RRT therapy.

We recommend the goal to be set as immediate and ongoing goals. The immediate goals for correcting electrolyte disturbance and academia should be providing bicarbonate or reducing hyperkalemia, controlling volume by removing fluid overload and improving hemodynamic stability. Ongoing goals including maintenance of fluid balance, promoting renal recovery, weaning from vasopressors, maintenance of acid–base and electrolyte balances and support of organ functions. Provide RRT to achieve the goals of electrolyte, acid–base, solute and fluid balances that will meet the patient's needs (not graded). [6].

*Fluid Balance*
The fluid management of CSA-AKI is also more complex and susceptible than other cause of AKI [33]. When the heart is impaired, the window of fluid protocol becomes narrower and the problem is that even small changes in fluid load may affect patient outcome. In particular, if we keep the patient too overloaded on fluid, the risk of complications such as myocardial or pulmonary edema,

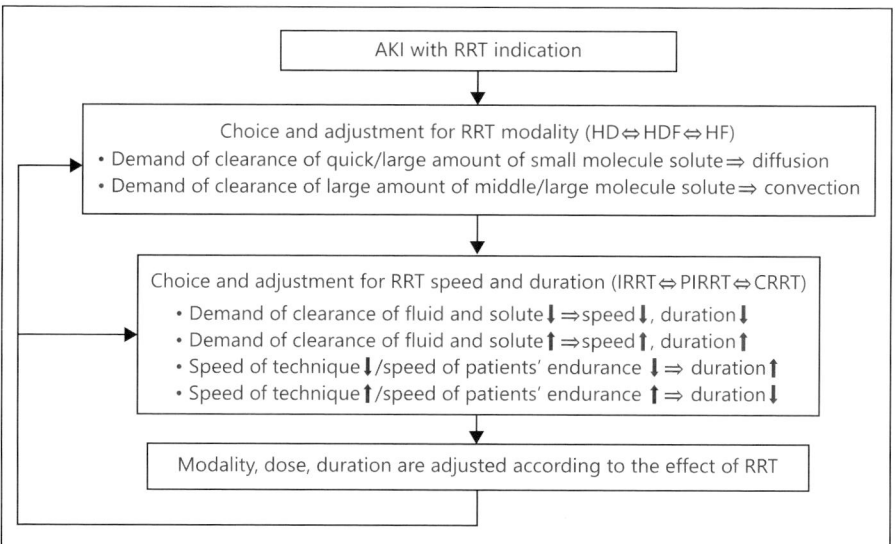

**Fig. 1.** Proposal for GDRRT. AKI = Acute kidney injury; RRT = renal replacement therapy; HD = hemodialysis; HDF = hemodiafiltration; HF = hemofiltration; IRRT = intermittent renal replacement therapy; PIRRT = prolonged intermittent renal replacement therapy; CRRT = continuous renal replacement therapy.

peripheral edema and organ congestion will obviously increase. But if we dehydrate the patient too much, the risk of complications such as hypotension, tachycardia and organ hypoperfusion may also increase. So the targets of fluid control may change depending on if the patient is under risk of different conditions. Sometimes, we have a very tight situation of optimal the fluid management, probably better according to the hemodynamic parameters.

## Conclusion

The incidence of CSA-AKI and mortality is unlikely to be significantly reduced by any one aspect of management due to its complex pathogenesis. Prevention and interventions of CSA-AKI requires a multimodal approach where both the premorbid condition of the patient and the particular idiosyncrasies of the cardiac surgical procedure itself are taken into account. Timely intervention requires early recognition of potential kidney injury. For now, RRT is the mainstay of supportive treatment for CSA-AKI patients. The prompt, judicious application of RRT is the key to improve outcomes. Potential favorable pharmacologic interventions include natriuretic peptides, such as nesiritide and use of dopamine agonists, such as fenoldopam may also help.

## References

1 Englberger L, Suri RM, Connolly HM, et al: Increased risk of acute kidney injury in patients undergoing tricuspid valve surgery. Eur J Cardiothorac Surg 2013;43:993–999.
2 Karkouti K, Wijeysundera DN, Yau TM, et al: Acute kidney injury after cardiac surgery: focus on modifiable risk factors. Circulation 2009;119:495–502.
3 Conlon PJ, Stafford-Smith M, White WD, et al: Acute renal failure following cardiac surgery. Nephrol Dial Transplant 1999;14:1158–1162.
4 Roy AK, Mc GC, Treacy C, et al: A Comparison of Traditional and Novel Definitions (RIFLE, AKIN, and KDIGO) of Acute Kidney Injury for the Prediction of Outcomes in Acute Decompensated Heart Failure. Cardio Renal Med 2013;3:26–37.
5 Shann KG, Likosky DS, Murkin JM, et al: An evidence-based review of the practice of cardiopulmonary bypass in adults: a focus on neurologic injury, glycemic control, hemodilution, and the inflammatory response. J Thorac Cardiovasc Surg 2006;132:283–290.
6 Kidney Disease: Improving Global Outcomes (KDIGO) Acute Kidney Injury Work Group. KDIGO clinical practice guideline for acute kidney injury. Kidney Inter 2012;2(suppl): 1–138.
7 Ghatanatti R, Teli A, Tirkey SS, Bhattacharya S, Sengupta G, Mondal A: Role of renal biomarkers as predictors of acute kidney injury in cardiac surgery. Asian Cardiovasc Thorac Ann 2014;22:234–241.
8 Rewa O, Bagshaw SM: Acute kidney injury-epidemiology, outcomes and economics. Nat Rev Nephrol 2014;10:193–207.
9 Chawla LS, Zhao Y, Lough FC, Schroeder E, Seneff MG, Brennan JM: Off-pump versus on-pump coronary artery bypass grafting outcomes stratified by preoperative renal function. J Am Soc Nephrol 2012;23:1389–1397.
10 Seabra VF, Alobaidi S, Balk EM, Poon AH, Jaber BL: Off-pump coronary artery bypass surgery and acute kidney injury: a meta-analysis of randomized controlled trials. Clin J Am Soc Nephrol 2010;5:1734–1744.
11 Ho KM, Morgan DJ: Meta-analysis of N-acetylcysteine to prevent acute renal failure after major surgery. Am J Kidney Dis 2009;53:33–40.
12 Liakopoulos OJ, Choi YH, Haldenwang PL, et al: Impact of preoperative statin therapy on adverse postoperative outcomes in patients undergoing cardiac surgery: a meta-analysis of over 30,000 patients. Eur Heart J 2008;29: 1548–1559.
13 Argalious M, Xu M, Sun Z, Smedira N, Koch CG: Preoperative statin therapy is not associated with a reduced incidence of postoperative acute kidney injury after cardiac surgery. Anesth Analg 2010;111:324–330.
14 Prowle JR, Calzavacca P, Licari E, et al: Pilot double-blind, randomized controlled trial of short-term atorvastatin for prevention of acute kidney injury after cardiac surgery. Nephrology (Carlton) 2012;17:215–224.
15 Fishbane S: N-acetylcysteine in the prevention of contrast-induced nephropathy. Clin J Am Soc Nephrol 2008;3:281–287.
16 DiMari J, Megyesi J, Udvarhelyi N, Price P, Davis R, Safirstein R: N-acetyl cysteine ameliorates ischemic renal failure. Am J Physiol 1997;272(3 Pt 2):F292–F298.
17 Nigwekar SU, Kandula P: N-acetylcysteine in cardiovascular-surgery-associated renal failure: a meta-analysis. Ann Thorac Surg 2009; 87:139–147.
18 Santana-Santos E, Gowdak LH, Gaiotto FA, et al: High dose of N-acetylcystein prevents acute kidney injury in chronic kidney disease patients undergoing myocardial revascularization. Ann Thorac Surg 2014;97:1617–1623.
19 Solomon R, Dauerman HL: Contrast-induced acute kidney injury. Circulation 2010;122: 2451–2455.
20 Brown JR, Block CA, Malenka DJ, O'Connor GT, Schoolwerth AC, Thompson CA: Sodium bicarbonate plus N-acetylcysteine prophylaxis: a meta-analysis. JACC Cardiovasc Interv 2009;2:1116–1124.
21 Tian ML, Hu Y, Yuan J, Zha Y: Efficacy and safety of perioperative sodium bicarbonate therapy for cardiac surgery-associated acute kidney injury: a meta-analysis. J Cardiovasc Pharmacol 2015;65:130–136.
22 Ranucci M, De Benedetti D, Bianchini C, et al: Effects of fenoldopam infusion in complex cardiac surgical operations: a prospective, randomized, double-blind, placebo-controlled study. Minerva Anestesiol 2010;76: 249–259.

23 Zangrillo A, Biondi-Zoccai GG, Frati E, et al: Fenoldopam and acute renal failure in cardiac surgery: a meta-analysis of randomized placebo-controlled trials. J Cardiothorac Vasc Anesth 2012;26:407–413.
24 Bove T, Zangrillo A, Guarracino F, et al: Effect of fenoldopam on use of renal replacement therapy among patients with acute kidney injury after cardiac surgery: a randomized clinical trial. JAMA 2014;312: 2244–2253.
25 Bove T, Calabro MG, Landoni G, et al: The incidence and risk of acute renal failure after cardiac surgery. J Cardiothorac Vasc Anesth 2004;18:442–445.
26 Bagshaw S M, Berthiaume L R, Delaney A, et al: Continuous versus intermittent renal replacement therapy for critically ill patients with acute kidney injury: a meta-analysis. Crit Care Med 2008;36:610–617.
27 Marsha MR ll, Creamer JM, Foster M, et al: Mortality rate comparison after switching from continuous to prolonged intermittent renal replacement for acute kidney injury in three intensive care units from different countries. Nephrol Dial Transplant 2011;26: 2169–2175.
28 Bellomo R, Cass A, Cole L, et al: Intensity of continuous renal-replacement therapy in critically ill patients. N Engl J Med 2009;361: 1627–1638.
29 Palevsky PM, Zhang JH, O'Connor TZ, et al: Intensity of renal support in critically ill patients with acute kidney injury. N Engl J Med 2008;359:7–20.
30 Evanson JA, Himmelfarb J, Wingard R, Knights S, Shyr Y, Schulman G, Ikizler TA, Hakim RM: Prescribed versus delivered dialysis in acute renal failure patients. Am J Kidney Dis 1998;32:731–738.
31 Mehta RL: Continuous renal replacement therapy in the critically ill patient. Kidney Int 2005;67:781–795.
32 Jiarui Xu, Xiaoqiang Ding, Yi Fang, et al: New, goal-directed approach to renal replacement therapy improves acute kidney injury treatment after cardiac surgery. J Cardiothorac Surg 2014;9:103.
33 Prowle JR, Chua HR, Bagshaw SM, et al: Clinical review: volume of fluid resuscitation and the incidence of acute kidney injury – a systematic review. Crit Care 2012;16:230.

Xiaoqiang Ding, MD, PhD
Division of Nephrology, Zhongshan Hospital
Shanghai Medical College, Fudan University
No.180 Fenglin Road
Shanghai 200032 (China)
E-Mail dingxiaoqiang2015@hotmail.com

# Author Index

Amdur, R.L.  55

Bagshaw, S.M.  106
Bellomo, R.  36
Brooks, C.H.  9

Chawla, L.S.  55
Cheungpasitporn, W.  73
Chopra, T.A.  9
Chuang, C.-L.  84

Ding, X.  VII, 1, 131

Fang, Y.  1, 131
Fuhrman, D.Y.  47

Goldstein, S.L.  121

Jiang, W.  131

Kashani, K.  73
Kellum, J.A.  47

Macedo, E.  24
Mårtensson, J.  36
Mehta, R.L.  24

Okusa, M.D.  9
Ostermann, M.  106

Palant, C.E.  55

Ricci, Z.  94, 121
Romagnoli, S.  94
Ronco, C.  VII, 94

Teng, J.  1, 131

Villa, G.  94

Wald, R.  106
Wang, Y.  1

Xu, J.  131

# Subject Index

N-Acetyl cysteine (NAC)
    cardiac surgery-associated acute kidney injury management 135
    contrast-induced acute kidney injury prevention 15, 16
Acute kidney injury, *see also specific causes*
    biomarkers, *see* Biomarkers, acute kidney injury
    definition 2, 3, 24
    fluid therapy, *see* Fluid therapy, acute kidney injury
    prevention 12–20
    renal recovery, *see* Renal recovery, acute kidney injury
    risk assessment 10–12
Acute kidney injury network, acute kidney injury criteria 2
Acute renal replacement therapy (ARRT)
    adequacy assessment 95–97
    anticoagulation 101–103
    cardiac surgery-associated acute kidney injury management
        cessation 138
        dose 138
        fluid therapy 139, 140
        goal-directed therapy 138–140
        modality 137
        timing 136, 137
    dose and recovery 32
    modality 100, 101
    outcome impact 107, 108
    overview 95, 97–99, 106, 107
    pediatric continuous renal replacement therapy
        epidemiology 121, 122
        extracorporeal membrane oxygenation patients 127, 128
        modalities 123–125
        technical aspects 125–128
        timing 122, 123
    timing of initiation
        clinical studies 112–115
        definition 109
        overview 99, 100
        prospects for study 116, 117
        rationale 109–112
        recommendations 115, 116
ALBIOS, *see* Albumin Italian Outcome Sepsis
Albumin Italian Outcome Sepsis (ALBIOS) 86
Allopurinol, acute kidney injury prevention 18
Angiotensin, acute kidney injury progression to chronic kidney disease 67
Aortic valve replacement, *see* Transcatheter aortic valve replacement
ARRT, *see* Acute renal replacement therapy

Biomarkers, acute kidney injury
    acute kidney injury progression to chronic kidney disease 68
    cardiac surgery-associated acute kidney injury 132

diagnosis 47–49
prognosis 49–52
therapy monitoring 52
BMP-7, see Bone morphogenetic protein-7
Bone morphogenetic protein-7 (BMP-7), acute kidney injury prevention 19, 20

CA-AKI, see Community-acquired acute kidney injury
Cardiac surgery-associated acute kidney injury (CSA-AKI)
biomarkers 132
contrast media insult 134
epidemiology 131
fluid therapy 139, 140
prevention 132–134
risk assessment 10, 11, 133
treatment 135–140
Cardio-Renal Pediatric Dialysis Emergency Machine (CARPEDIEM) 125
CARPEDIEM, see Cardio-Renal Pediatric Dialysis Emergency Machine
CHEST, see Crystalloid versus Hydroxyethyl Starch Trial
China, acute kidney injury features 6
Chronic kidney disease (CKD), acute kidney injury progression
biomarkers 68
epidemiology 56–62
hypertension following injury 68
overview 5, 27, 28
pathophysiology 62–68
prospects for study 69
risk factors 61
survival 57–59
CI-AKI, see Contrast-induced acute kidney injury
CKD, see Chronic kidney disease
Community-acquired acute kidney injury (CA-AKI) 4
Continuous renal replacement therapy, see Acute renal replacement therapy
Continuous venovenous hemofiltration, see Acute renal replacement therapy

Contrast-induced acute kidney injury (CI-AKI)
cardiac surgery-associated acute kidney injury 134
mechanisms and risk factors 12, 13
prevention
N-acetyl cysteine 15, 16
isotonic saline use 14, 15
low-risk contrast agent use 13, 14
risk assessment 12
Crystalloid versus Hydroxyethyl Starch Trial (CHEST) 86
CSA-AKI, see Cardiac surgery-associated acute kidney injury

Dopamine, acute kidney injury prevention 18

ECMO, see Extracorporeal membrane oxygenation
EHR, see Electronic health record
Electronic health record (EHR)
automated acute kidney injury alerts
algorithm 78
challenges with serum creatinine and urine output criteria 79
rationale 74–77
sensitivity and specificity 79, 80
historical perspective 73–75
prospects 81
research applications 80, 81
risk stratification for acute kidney injury 80
Epigenetics, acute kidney injury progression to chronic kidney disease 64
Extracorporeal membrane oxygenation (ECMO), pediatric continuous renal replacement therapy 127, 128

Fenoldopam
acute kidney injury prevention 18
cardiac surgery-associated acute kidney injury management 136
Fluid therapy, acute kidney injury
cardiac surgery-associated acute kidney injury management 139, 140

colloids 85, 86
crystalloids 86, 87
overview 84, 85
rationale 87, 88
responsiveness in critically ill patients
    measurement 88, 89
    prediction 89, 90

HA-AKI, *see* Hospital-acquired acute kidney injury
Hepatocyte growth factor (HGF), acute kidney injury progression to chronic kidney disease biomarker 68
Hepcidin, acute kidney injury prevention 20
HGF, *see* Hepatocyte growth factor
HIF, *see* Hypoxia-inducible factor
Hospital-acquired acute kidney injury (HA-AKI) 4
Hypertension, acute kidney injury association 68
Hypoxia-inducible factor (HIF)
    acute kidney injury progression to chronic kidney disease 65, 67
    targeting in acute kidney injury prevention 19

IGF-I, *see* Insulin-like growth factor-I
IGFBP7
    prognostic biomarker 49, 50, 52
    therapeutic intervention monitoring 52
Incidence, AKI 1, 3, 4
Insulin-like growth factor-I (IGF-I), acute kidney injury management 17

KDIGO, *see* Kidney Disease: Improving Global Outcomes
Kidney Disease: Improving Global Outcomes (KDIGO), acute kidney injury criteria 2, 3, 47, 48, 115

Mannitol, acute kidney injury prevention 18
Mesenchymal stem cell (MSC), acute kidney injury prevention 20, 21

MicroRNA, acute kidney injury progression to chronic kidney disease 64
Mitiquinone mesylate (MitoQ), acute kidney injury prevention 17
MitoQ, *see* Mitiquinone mesylate
Mortality, acute kidney injury 5, 9, 36
MSC, *see* Mesenchymal stem cell

NAC, *see* N-Acetyl cysteine
Neutrophil gelatinase-associated lipocalin (NGAL)
    acute kidney injury progression to chronic kidney disease biomarker 68
    diagnostic biomarker 48
    prognostic biomarker 49
    septic acute kidney injury pathophysiology 38, 39
NGAL, *see* Neutrophil gelatinase-associated lipocalin

Peritoneal dialysis, *see* Acute renal replacement therapy
Peroxisome proliferator-activated receptor-α (PPARα), agonists for acute kidney injury prevention 18
PPARα, *see* Peroxisome proliferator-activated receptor-α

Randomized Evaluation of Normal versus Augmented Level Replacement Therapy (RENAL) 122
Rasburicase, acute kidney injury prevention 18
Renal recovery, acute kidney injury
    assessment 25, 26, 33
    care process 31, 32
    chronic kidney disease progression 5, 27, 28
    determinants 28–30
    epidemiologic data 26, 27
    modifiable risk factors 30, 31
    renal replacement therapy dose and recovery 32
Renal replacement therapy, *see* Acute renal replacement therapy

RENAL, *see* Randomized Evaluation of Normal versus Augmented Level Replacement Therapy
RIFLE, acute kidney injury criteria  2, 24

SAFE, *see* Saline versus Albumin Fluid Evaluation
Saline versus Albumin Fluid Evaluation (SAFE)  86
Septic acute kidney injury
    overview  36, 37
    pathophysiology
        cellular activation  37–39
        cellular hibernation  39
        cellular suicide  39, 40
        tubular injury and impaired glomerular filtration  40–42
    renal hemodynamics  42, 43
    therapeutic targets  41, 42
SS-31, acute kidney injury prevention  17, 19
Statins
    acute kidney injury prevention  18
    cardiac surgery-associated acute kidney injury management  135

TAVR, *see* Transcatheter aortic valve replacement
TIMP-2, *see* Tissue inhibitor of metalloproteinase-2
Tissue inhibitor of metalloproteinase-2 (TIMP-2)
    prognostic biomarker  49, 50, 52
    therapeutic intervention monitoring  52
Transcatheter aortic valve replacement (TAVR), acute kidney injury  11

VAD, *see* Ventricular assist device
Vascular endothelial growth factor (VEGF), acute kidney injury progression to chronic kidney disease  65
VEGF, *see* Vascular endothelial growth factor
Ventricular assist device (VAD), acute kidney injury  12